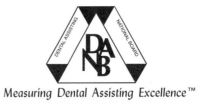

Measuring Dental Assisting Excellence™

DANB's
Glossary of Dental Assisting Terms
Second Edition

A guide to applied practical & clinical dental terminology

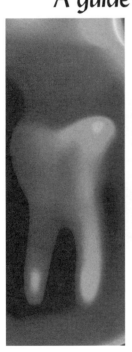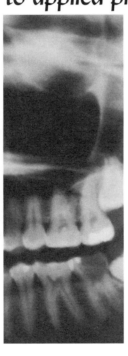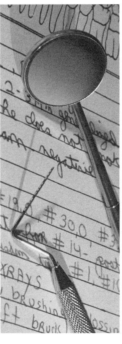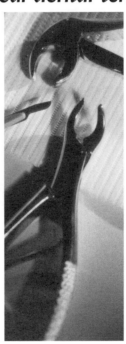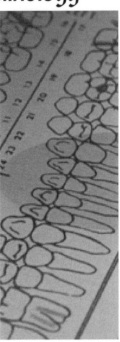

Cynthia C. Durley, MEd, MBA
Liz Koch, MA, MPH
Kathy Brown, CDA, RDA, BES
Dawn Capper, BS

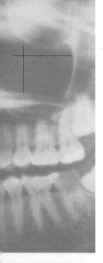
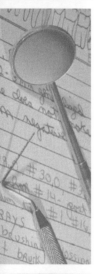
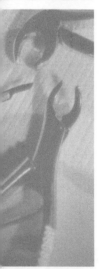
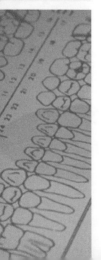

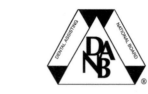

Measuring Dental Assisting Excellence™

© 2005 The Dental Assisting National Board, Inc.®
676 N. St. Clair, Suite 1880
Chicago, Illinois 60611
1-800-FOR-DANB
www.danb.org
danbmail@danb.org

ISBN: 0-9720066-7-2

TABLE OF CONTENTS

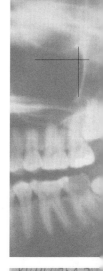
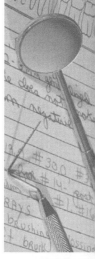
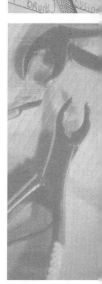
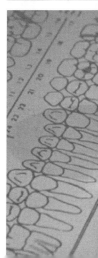

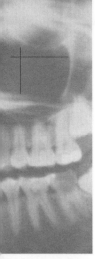
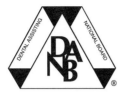
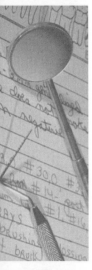

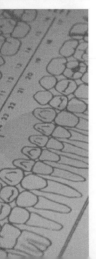

The Dental Assisting National Board, Inc. (DANB) is a non-profit corporation whose mission is to promote the public good by providing credentialing services to the dental community.

DANB measures the success of this mission by providing:

- a properly governed, financially secure and administratively sound organization
- valid dental assisting credentialing exams
- dental assisting recertification process integrity
- visible, valuable, accessible DANB credentials
- other testing services for groups within the dental community, as deemed appropriate
- information services for the oral healthcare community related to dental assisting credentialing and recertification

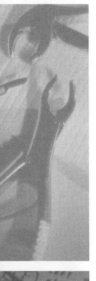

DANB is a member of the National Organization for Competency Assurance (NOCA). The National Commission For Certifying Agencies (NCCA), a NOCA Commission with responsibility for evaluating credentialing programs, has accredited DANB national certification exam programs, (CDA, COA, CDPMA and COMSA), including DANB component exams (RHS, ICE, GC and OA) and found DANB programs meet NCCA's highest standards, thus helping to assure validity, reliability, and objectivity in the testing process.

INTRODUCTION

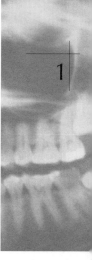

The Dental Assisting National Board, Inc. (DANB) congratulates you on your accomplishments. You are an important part of the vibrant and challenging career of dental assisting. We commend you on your commitment to excellence through DANB Certification.

DANB has been the recognized national leader in dental assisting certification for more than 50 years. Through DANB credentialing programs, assistants demonstrate their knowledge and commitment to practice excellence in all aspects of assisting from patient care to infection control, and from radiation health and safety to front office operations. The Certified Dental Assistant (CDA®), Certified Orthodontic Assistant (COA®), and Certified Dental Practice Management Administrator (CDPMA®) certifications allow you entrance into a select group of more than 30,000 currently certified assistants throughout the world.

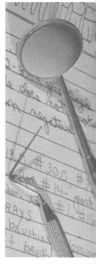

As dentistry and the dental assisting profession continues to progress and develop, precise understanding of dental terminology is essential in communication with patients, employers, and dental care providers. Dental vocabulary is many times the only means to truly express data, concepts and procedures, thus creating a successful interchange of ideas among the entire dental team—the foundation for effective communication and professional relationships with patients and colleagues.

DANB's Glossary of Dental Assisting Terms consists of many practical and clinical terms with definitions that are relevant to DANB administered examinations and the dental assisting profession. The *Glossary* is a learning resource for examination preparation. It is also a valuable tool for dental assistants new to the profession, dental office management personnel, dental assisting students, as well as experienced dental assistants, dental assisting educators, clinicians, and employers.

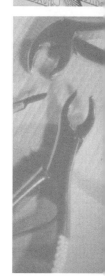

The intent of this book is to provide definitions to dental terms with an emphasis on clinical use of these terms, and to provide a broad knowledge of the professional language. Some dental terms may have a variety of connotations from general to specialized dentistry. The aim is not to represent all the meanings of each term but to present with simplicity and clarity the most common definitions used in practice and presented in educational dental assisting programs.

DANB's Glossary of Dental Assisting Terms is not a comprehensive publication with all possible dental-related words that you would find in a medical/dental dictionary, however. It is a dynamic publication, with entries reflecting more difficult concepts tested on DANB examinations. DANB will update the *Glossary* regularly to add new words found on DANB examinations to future *Glossary* editions.

In addition to the body of the *Glossary,* you will find two appendices:

Appendix A is a listing of relevant associations, organizations, and governmental agencies, including its founding year, headquarters location, and purpose. This appendix is limited to those associations, organizations, or agencies referenced within a DANB examination, related to measurement issues, or which you and your colleagues may encounter while carrying out your professional responsibilities. Many entries in Appendix A have been reprinted with permission of the Joint Commission on Accreditation of Healthcare Organizations (JCAHO), as published in JCAHO's *Lexikon,* 1998.

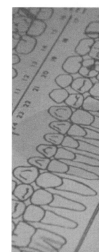

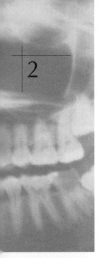

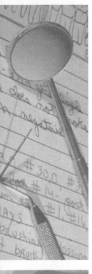

Appendix B is a listing of State Dental Board street addresses, phone and fax numbers, contact persons, and e-mail addresses and/or web sites where available, for all 50 states plus the District of Columbia.

In tandem with *The DANB Review*, DANB believes this publication will aid you as you prepare for DANB exams and continue in the field of dental assisting. (Please note that purchasing this *Glossary* or any other publication is not required to pass a DANB exam, nor do they guarantee success.)

DANB's Glossary of Dental Assisting Terms was developed in consultation with DANB's Board of Directors. DANB is very appreciative of the contributions of the individuals listed below who serve on the DANB Board of Directors' Exam Program Committee, which oversees the content in DANB exam review publications.

We hope you find this study guide helpful in preparing for your DANB exam. Best wishes for a prosperous and successful future!

Cindy Durley, MEd,MBA
Executive Director, DANB

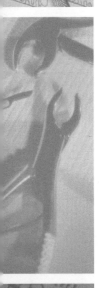

DANB's Glossary of Dental Assisting Terms was compiled and edited by:

Kathy Brown, BES, CDA, RDA
Assistant Director, Test Administration, Dental Assisting National Board, Inc.

Cynthia C. Durley, MEd, MBA
Executive Director, Dental Assisting National Board, Inc.

Elizabeth Koch, MA, MPH
Director, Test Administration, Dental Assisting National Board, Inc.

Dawn Capper, BS
Director, Marketing & Communications, Dental Assisting National Board, Inc.

DANB Board of Directors' Exam Program Committee
Carla Schneider, CDA, RDA
Brenda Fell, CDA, CDPMA
Paul Stubbs, DDS
Thomas Harrison, DDS

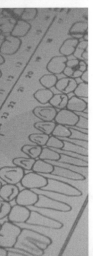

REFERENCES

Dietz, E., *Dental Office Management*, Delmar Thompson Learning, Albany, NY, 2000, (800) 477-3692

Dofka, C.M., Dental Terminology, Delmar Thompson Learning, Albany, NY, 2000, (800) 477-3692

Finkbeiner, B.L. and Johnson, C.S., *Comprehensive Dental Assisting, A Clinical Approach*, C.V. Mosby, St. Louis, MO, 1995, (800) 325-4177

Miles, D., Van Dis., Jensen, C., and Ferretti, A., *Radiographic Imaging for Dental Auxiliaries*, W. B. Saunders, Philadelphia, PA, 2001, (800) 325-4177

Mosby's Dental Dictionary, published by C.V. Mosby (An Affiliate of Elsevier), St. Louis, MO, 2004, (800) 325-4177

Novak, D.E., Contemporary Dental Assisting, C.V. Mosby, St. Louis, MO, 2001, (800) 325-4177

Phinney, D.J. and Halstead, J.H., *Dental Assisting a Comprehensive Approach*, Delmar Thompson Learning, Albany, NY, 2000, (800) 477-3692

Physician's Desk Reference, Thompson Medical Economics Company, Montvale, NJ, 2002 (201) 358-7200

Robinson, D. and Bird, D., *Essentials of Dental Assisting, Third Edition*, W. B. Saunders, Philadelphia, PA, 2001, (800) 325-4177

Robinson, D. and Bird, D., *Torres' and Ehrlich's Modern Dental Assisting, Sixth Edition*, W. B. Saunders, Philadelphia, PA, 2002, (800) 325-4177

Tabers Cyclopedic Medical Dictionary, 18th Edition, F.A. Davis Company, Philadelphia, PA, 1997, (800) 323-3555

www.handhygiene.org

Zwemer, T.J., *Boncher's Clinical Dental Terminology, Fourth Edition*, C.V. Mosby, St. Louis, MO, 1993, (800) 325-4177

A list of additional exam resources can be found on the DANB website at www.danb.org or in any of the DANB Exam Candidate Guides, available by calling 1-800-FOR-DANB.

DANB welcomes comments and suggestions regarding the *Glossary*. If there are any terms you don't see in this Glossary and would like us to include in the next edition, please send your comments and suggestions to examdev@danb.org or Dental Assistant, DANB, 676 N. St. Clair, Suite 1880, Chicago, IL 60611.

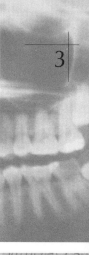
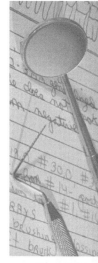
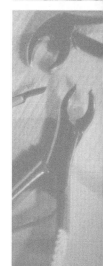
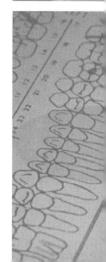

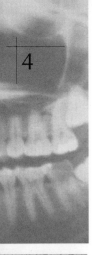

4

ROOT WORDS

A root word is the foundation of a word to which prefixes and suffixes may be added. Following are many common root words used in dental terminology:

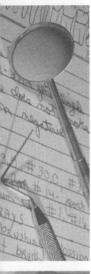

aden	gland
aer	air
alba	white
arthr	joint
bio	life
blast	process of budding (cell division)
bucc	check
cantho	angle such as the corner of the eye
carcin	cancer
cardi	heart
ceph	head
cervi	neck
cheil	lip (mouth)
chondro	cartilage
cost	rib
crani	head
cyto	cell
denti	tooth
derma	skin
disto	away from the middle
erythro	red
gastr	stomach
gloss	tongue
idio	relationship to self
labi	lip
lacto	milk
linea	line
lingo	tongue
leuk	white
mental	chin
mesio	towards the middle
naso	nose
nephro	kidney
neuro	nerve
odont	tooth
pedo	child
psycho	mind
renal	kidney
somato	body
therm	temperature; hot
vaso	vessel

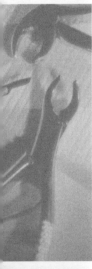

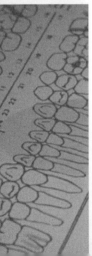

Prefixes

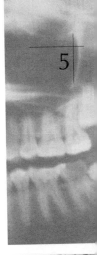

A prefix is a word division that is attached to the beginning of a term to alter the meaning by adding quantity, condition, location and size. Following are many common prefixes used in dental terminology:

a	without
ab	away from; negative
ad/ac	toward; increase
ante	before; preceding
anti	effectiveness against
auto	self
bi	two
bio	life; living
co	with; together
con	with; together
com	with; together
contra	opposite
cyan	blue
cyst	sac or bladder
cyto	cell
di	twice; double
dia	through; apart; across
dys	faulty
e	without
endo	within
ex	away from
fore	toward the front
gnath	jaw
histo	tissue
hyper	abnormally high; more than
hypo	abnormally low; less than
infra	under; beneath
inter	between
intra	inside; within
mal	ill or bad
neo	new
osteo	bone
patho	disease
peri	around
pre	before; in front of
pro	in front of; forward
pseudo	false
pyo	pus
retro	back; behind
semi	half
sub	under; below; almost
syn	with; together
super	above; beyond; upper; excessive
supra	above
trans	across; through
tri	three
uni	one
vaso	blood vessel

Suffixes

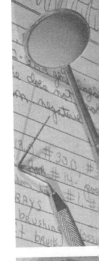

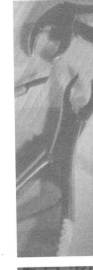

A suffix is attached to the end of a term to describe or qualify the word meaning or alter the meaning by adding quantity, condition, procedure or state of being. Following are many common suffixes used in dental terminology:

al	expressing relationship; pertaining to or concerning
algia	pain
blast	grow; sprout
cele	protrusion; swelling; enlarged space
cide	kill
clast	break
ectomy	remove
esthesia	feeling; sensation
gen	relating to production by a gene; the beginning
genic	relating to production by a gene; the beginning
geny	relating to production by a gene; the beginning
ia	condition; state of being
ic	denoting science, practice, or treatment
ism	characteristic of behavior
ist	specialist in
itis	inflammation
ize	to cause to be
lysis	breaking up; dissolving
ologist	specialist in the study of
ology	studies or concepts
oma	indicates tumor; swelling
osis	condition or state of being
otomy	surgical incision; partial removal
ous	pertaining to; composed of; expressing material
plasty	surgically shaped
pnea	breathing; breath
rhea	flow; discharge
sion	condition; state
stasis	stop; stand still
tic	showing relationship to
trophy	development; growth
um	plural ending added to nouns
us	singular ending added to nouns

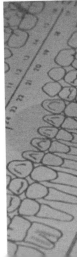

ABBREVIATIONS COMMONLY USED IN PRESCRIPTION WRITING

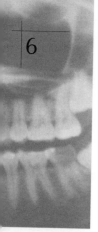
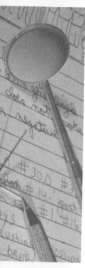
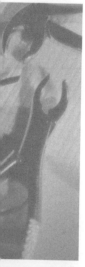
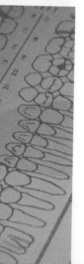

a.a.	of each
a.c.	before meals
a.d.	to; up to
ad lib	as often as is wanted
a.m.	morning
aq	water
b.i.d.	twice a day
cap	capsule
god	every other day
h	hour
h.s.	at bedtime
tab	tablet
t.i.d.	three times a day
liq	liquid
ml	milliliter
n.p.o.	nothing by mouth
p.c.	after meals
po (per os)	by mouth
p.r.n.	as occasion arises; as needed
q.	each
q.d.	daily
q.h.s.	every night at bedtime
q.2.h.	every 2 hours
q.3.h.	(q3h) every three hours
q.4.h.	every four hours
q.8.h.	every eight hours
q.i.d.	four times a day
Rx	prescription
Sig.	Write; let it be written
stat	immediately
Ô	one tablespoon
T. tbs	tablespoon
t, tsp	teaspoon
i	one
ii	two
iii	three

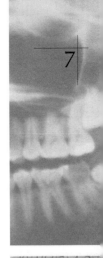

ADA	American Dental Association
ADA	Americans with Disabilities Act
ADAA	American Dental Assistants Association
ADHA	American Dental Hygenists Association
AIDS	acquired immunodeficiency syndrome
ALARA	as low as reasonably achievable
ANSI	American National Standards Institute
ANUG	acute necrotizing ulcerative gingivitis
BBP	bloodborne pathogens
BI	biological indicator
BOD	Board of Dentistry (aka: Board of Dental Examiners)
BWX	bitewing radiographs (x-rays)
CDC	Centers for Disease Control and Prevention
CEJ	cementoenamel junction
cfu/ml	colony-forming units per milliliter of water
CNS	central nervous system
COPD	chronic obstructive pulmonary disease
CPR	cardiopulmonary resuscitation
CRE	central ray entry
CT	computerized tomography
DDS	Doctor of Dental Surgery
DHCP	dental healthcare personnel
DHCW	dental healthcare worker
DMD	Doctor of Medical Dentistry
DPA	Dental Practice Act
DPM	Dental Practice Management
DUWL	dental unit waterlines
EOB	explanation of benefits
EPA	Environmental Protection Agency
FDA	Food and Drug Administration
FMX	full mouth x-rays
GC	General Chairside Exam (DANB)
HA	horizontal angle
HAV	hepatitus A virus
HBV	hepatitis B virus
HCAI	healthcare associated infections
HCV	hepatitis C virus
HDV	hepatitis D virus
HEV	hepatitis E virus
HGV	hepatitis G virus
HIPAA	Health Insurance Portability & Accountability Act
HIV	human immunodeficiency virus
HMO	Health Maintenance Organization
HVE	high volume evacuation
ICE	Infection Control Exam (DANB)
ICO	infection control officer

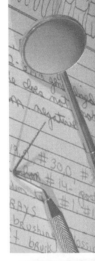

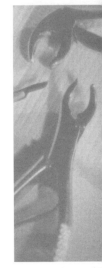

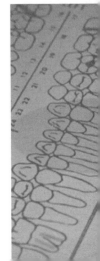

ACRONYMS *(CONTINUED)*

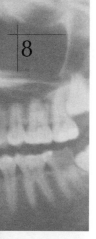
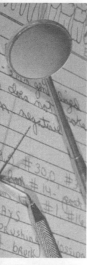
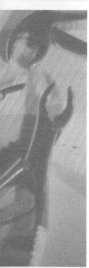
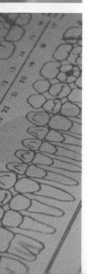

JCAHO	Joint Commission on Accreditation of Healthcare Organizations
kVp	kilovoltage peak
mA	milliamperage
MPD	maximum permissible dose
MRI	magnetic resonance imaging
MSDS	Material Safety Data Sheet
NCRP	National Council on Radiation Protection and Measurement
NNIS	national nosocomial infection systems
N$_2$O	nitrous oxide oxygen relative analgesia
NSF	nonsufficient funds
O$_2$	oxygen
OFD	object to film distance
OHI	oral hygiene instruction
OPIM	other potentially infectious materials
OSAP	Organization for Safety and Asepsis Procedures
OSHA	Occupational Safety and Health Administration
OTC	over-the-counter
PA	periapical radiographs
PDR	Physician's Desk Reference
PEP	post exposure prophylaxis
PHI	protected health information
PID	position indicating device (cone)
PPE	personal protection equipment
ppm	parts per million
PPO	Preferred Provider Organization
psi	pounds per square inch
QC	quality control
rad	radiation absorbed dose
rbc	red blood cells
RCT	root canal treatment/therapy
Rem	radiation equivalent man
RHS	Radiation Health and Safety Exam (DANB)
Rx	prescription
SARS	severe acute respiratory syndrome
SBE	subacute bacterial endocarditis
STD	sexually transmitted disease
TB	tuberculosis
TFD	target to film distance
TMJ/TMD	temporomandibular joint/dysfunction
TOD	target to object distance
Tx	treatment
UCR	usual, customary, and reasonable
VA	vertical angle
wbc	white blood cells
wnl	within normal limits
ZOE	zinc oxide-eugenol

TERMS

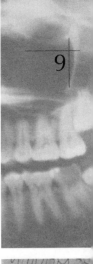

abandonment	failure to continue treatment on a patient without prior notice
abdominal thrust	see Heimlich maneuver
abfraction	a "V" or wedge-shaped defect at the cementoenamel junction caused by repeated clenching or grinding
abrasion	abnormal wearing away of tooth structure from incorrect brushing technique or other mechanical means
abrasive particles	material that cuts or grinds a surface, leaving grooves; used to remove soft deposits and stain or polish surfaces
abrasive strip	thin strip of plastic, metal or similar material, with an abrasive material bonded onto it used to contour and polish proximal surfaces of restorations
abscess, periapical	acute infection located at the apex of a nonvital (not living) tooth
abscess, periodontal	acute infection located at the base of a periodontal pocket
absorb	to take in; to retain (as with radiation exposure); to soak up liquids
absorbent	capable of taking up; usually refers to fluids; may also refer to taking in ionizing radiation or ultraviolet (UV) rays
abutment tooth/teeth	tooth/teeth or implant used to support a fixed multiple unit bridge or a removable partial denture
accelerator	catalyst; when added to a mixture speeds up the setting time of alginate, cement, gypsum products, etc.
accessible	easily obtained; easily entered
account ledger	record of services, charges (debits), and payments (credits) for an account
accounts payable	financial obligations or money owed by a practice for goods or services
accounts receivable	money owed to a practice from patients for services rendered
accurate	correct or precise

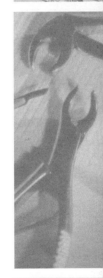

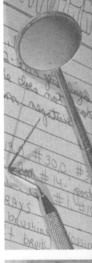

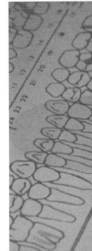

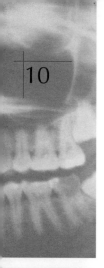

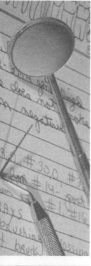

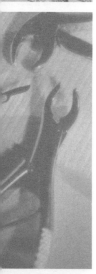

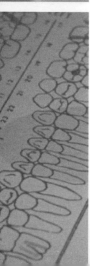

a

acetic acid	refers to vinegar; solvent used to remove calculus from removable prosthesis
acid etchant	see etchant
acidic	corrosive; consisting of an acid, not a base; having a pH greater than 7
acrylic	synthetic resin used to fabricate provisional restorations, dentures, removable partials, retainers, etc.
acquired immunodeficiency syndrome (AIDS)	disorder of the immune system that destroys the body's ability to fight infection; viral bloodborne sexually transmitted disease
activator	removable orthodontic appliance that expands the width of the maxillary arch
acupressure	an Oriental treatment for pain or illness in which pressure is applied to the skin at (meridian) points determined to be beneficial according to the condition being treated
acupuncture	an Oriental treatment for pain or illness in which fine needles are inserted through the skin at (meridian) points determined to be beneficial according to the condition being treated
acute	severe or intense; sudden or immediate; coming on quickly, lasting a short-term, but with severe symptoms (i.e., acute symptoms, as contrasted with chronic symptoms); active
acute necrotizing ulcerative gingivitis (ANUG)	a painful, progressive bacterial infection classified as a form of gingivitis and associated with decreased resistance to infection under conditions such as poor nutrition, extreme stress, or lack of adequate rest
ADA	American Dental Association; see Appendix A
ADA	acronym for Americans with Disabilities Act
ADAA	American Dental Assistants Association; see Appendix A
adaptation	change made to a material, process, or individual to make it suitable to the current situation
addiction	psychological or physical dependence on a habit forming substance
ADHA	American Dental Hygenists Association; see Appendix A
adhere	to join together or attach to
adhesion	binding together of two or more substances

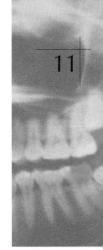

adhesive	material used to improve retention between two components
adjacent	next to
administer	to give or apply
administrative controls	the Occupational Safety and Health Administration (OSHA) identifies these as policies and procedures used to reduce the risk of an employee's exposure to pathogenic organisms
adrenaline	hormone involved in regulating glycogen (sugar) breakdown and synthesis; another name for epinephrine which is the principle blood-pressure raising hormone; used as a vasoconstrictor in controlling hemorrages of the skin and dilates (opens up) the bronchioles in bronchial asthma
adversely	acting in opposition to; moving in an opposite direction; affecting negatively
aerosol inhalation	ingestion of aerosolized particles through the nasal passages (nose) or oral cavity into the lungs
aerosolization	atomized particles suspended in air
agitate	move with sudden force; to stir
AIDS	see acquired immunodeficiency syndrome
air abrasion	process that removes minute amounts of tooth structure during cavity preparation through the use of alumina and high air pressure
air compressor	equipment that produces compressed air used to run handpieces and air/water syringes
air/water syringe	equipment that emits a stream of air or water, or a spray of air and water
ala	refers to the corner of the nose; often used in dental radiology (along with the tragus of the ear) to help in positioning the head
ALARA principal (as low as reasonably achievable)	radiographic principle that dictates the use of every method available to reduce radiation exposure to the patient in order to minimize risks and adverse consequences of ionizing radiation
alcohol	organic chemical once used for disinfection but no longer recommended because its property of rapid evaporation renders it ineffective
alcohol-based (waterless) handrub	an alcohol-containing medium developed for application to the hands to reduce the number of microorganisms on the hands; such preparations usually contain 60% to 95% ethanol or isopropanol

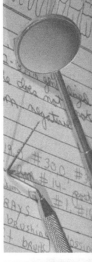

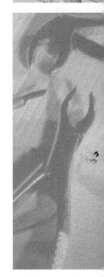

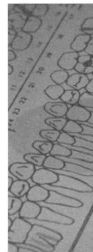

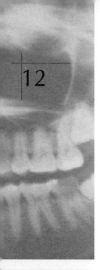

a

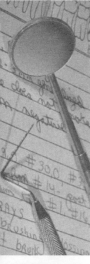

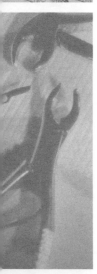

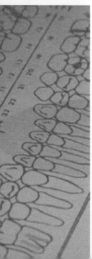

alginate	irreversible hydrocolloid impression material used for the fabrication of study casts, opposing models, custom trays, bleaching trays, mouth guards, etc.
alkaline	basic; non-acidic; having a pH less than 7
allergic reaction	reaction of the body to allergens, often initially characterized by itching, redness of the skin, hives, respiratory distress; may progress to a life-threatening state (see anaphylaxis) if untreated
allergen	substance that produces allergic reactions
alloy	combination of two or more metals but not mercury; term is sometimes incorrectly used interchangeably with amalgam; can refer to silver-based as well as gold-based metals
alumina	aluminum oxide polishing agent
aluminum filter	disk(s) of aluminum (usually about 0.5 mm thick) placed in the pathway of the x-ray beam used to filter out the long (non-penetrating) wavelengths from the x-ray beam
alveolar bone	bone that forms the tooth socket and supports the tooth in its position in the jaw
alveolar crest	most coronal portion of the alveolar bone; where two cortical bones join between each tooth
alveolar mucosa	thin, loosely attached tissue covering the alveolar bone
alveolar process	an elevation of bone on the maxilla and mandible that forms the arches
alveolar ridge	bony ridge of the maxilla and mandible that contains the sockets of the teeth and gives support to the teeth
alveolitis (dry socket)	condition/inflammation caused by a loss of the blood clot in a socket after an extraction
alveoloplasty	surgical shaping and smoothing of the margins of the tooth socket (alveolar bone) after extraction of a tooth, usually done in preparation for the placement of a prosthesis
alveolus	bone that surrounds the root of the tooth; the socket
amalgam	combination of two or more metals, one of which is mercury; blend of a powdered metal alloy and mercury to produce a restorative material
amalgamation	process of mixing amalgam; trituration
amalgamator	equipment that mixes amalgam and composite

ameloblasts	enamel forming cells
Americans with Disabilities Act (ADA)	federal law passed in 1990 that requires that people with disabilities be granted equal employment, access to public services and public accommodations, and goods and services; includes provision of telecommunication services to the hearing and speech impaired
amoxicillin	a penicillin-based antibiotic with a broadened spectrum of antimicrobial effectiveness
ampicillin	a penicillin-based antibiotic with a broadened spectrum of antimicrobial effectiveness
ampule	small glass vial used as a container for injectable solutions
amyl nitrate	vasodilator often prescribed for anginal pain
analgesic	drug that relieves pain
anaphylactic shock	immediate, severe, and sometimes fatal allergic reaction to a protein substance to which a patient is sensitized; symptoms may include feeling ill, nausea, shortness of breath, heart arrhythmia, drop in blood pressure, and loss or consciousness
anaphylaxis	systemic allergic reaction characterized by sudden collapse, shock, and respiratory and circulatory failure after an injection of an allergen
anatomical crown	portion of a tooth that is covered by enamel and extends from the root to the incisal or occusal edge
anatomy	science of the form, structure, and composition of an organism and the association of its parts
anemic	lacking the proper amount of red blood cells or volume of blood; low iron content of blood, resulting in fatigue
anesthesia	agents that cause loss of feeling, with or without loss of consciousness

Category

general– unconscious sedation

local– restricted to a specific area of the body/mouth and usually consisting of infiltration and block techniques

topical– direct placement by gel, liquid or patch to cause surface loss of sensation of mucous membranes

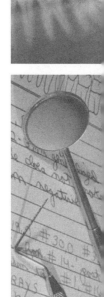

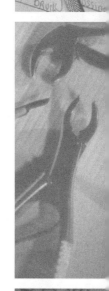

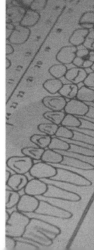

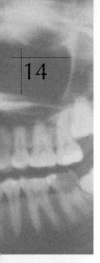

a

anesthesia *(continued)*	Mechanism
	block– anesthetic solution is injected near a main nerve trunk such as the inferior alveolar nerve of the mandibular arch
	infiltration– anesthetic solution is injected into the gingival and alveolar tissues of the maxillary arch near small terminal nerve branches for absorption
anesthetic	agent injected, inhaled or applied topically to reduce or eliminate feeling pain or sensation
anesthetic cartridge or carpule	glass cylinder that holds a premeasured quantity of sterile solution, such as an anesthetic solution
anesthetize	to induce anesthesia
angina pectoris	pain or pressure in the chest, caused by inadequate oxygen to the heart, which may radiate into the jaw, neck, or arm
angle of the mandible	where the body of the mandible meets the ramus
Angle's classification	classification of occlusion and malocclusion defined by Edward Angle in the late1800's; distinguished by the type of relationship between maxillary and mandibular first molars
angulation	direction of the primary beam of radiation to the radiographic film
	horizontal– beam is directed through the contacts of the teeth
	vertical– angulation that is perpendicular to the film and the long axis of the teeth
ankyloglossia	tongue tied
ankylosis	condition where tooth, cementum or dentin is fused to the bone limiting or preventing movement of a tooth
anneal	process of heating metal to a temperature below melting, holding it at that temperature for a length of time to keep the metal from becoming brittle; quickly heating gold foil just before being placed in order to remove surface impurities and oxides
anomaly	any deviation from normal
antecubital fossa	area on the inside of the elbow that may be used for the administration of intravenous solutions
anterior	toward the front of the mouth

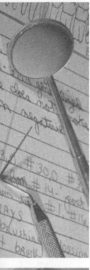
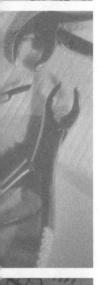
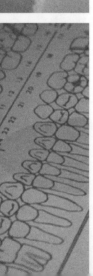

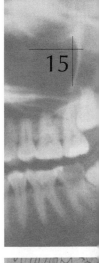

anterior band removing pliers	instrument used to shear or remove maxillary (upper) and mandibular (lower) anterior orthodontic bands
antibiotic	drug used to inhibit growth of or destroy microorganisms
antibodies	disease fighting protein produced by the body in response to an antigen
anticariogenic	against caries (cavity) production or generation
anticoagulant	agent that prevents/decreases coagulation (clotting) of blood
anticonvulsant	agent that prevents/controls convulsions or seizures
antidepressant	drug used to prevent or relieve depression
antigen	agent that activates the production of antibodies
antihistamine	agent that counteracts the body's production of histamine during an allergic reaction
antimicrobial	agent that prevents the development or action of microbes
antimicrobial agents	chemicals that inhibit growth of organisms; includes handscrubs or mouthwashes
antimicrobial soap	soap (detergent) containing an antiseptic agent
antipyretic	fever reducing drug
antiretraction valve	valve that is placed on lines that emit water to prevent reverse flow of fluids from patients into the lines of handpieces and evacuation systems
antiseptic agent	substance applied to the skin to reduce the number of microorganisms. (i.e.: alcohols, chlorexidine, chlorine, hexachlorophene, iodophors, chloroxylenol (PCMX), quaternary ammonium compounds, and triclosan)
antiseptic handwash	washing hands with water and soap or other detergents containing an antiseptic agent
anode	portion of the x-ray tube head that produces a positive charge
ANSI	American National Standards Institute; see Appendix A
ANUG	see acute necrotizing ulcerative gingivitis
anxiety	feeling of tension, dread, fear or distress over a real or imagined threat to one's mental or physical well-being
aperture	opening or hole

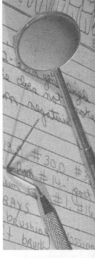

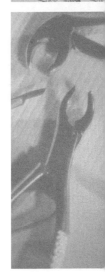

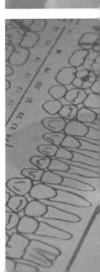

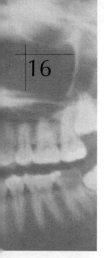

a

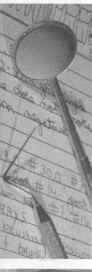

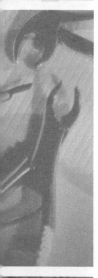

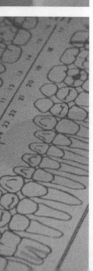

apex	tip of the root of a tooth
aphthous ulcers	cancer sore; an ulcer that forms secondary to herpes simplex; a shallow ulcer with an irregular, red border and a yellow-gray base
apical	pertaining to the end of the root of a tooth
apical foramen	opening in the apex of a tooth to allow entrance for nerve and blood vessels
apicoectomy	surgical removal of the apex of a tooth and associated infection
apnea	disruption in the breathing process characterized by a gradual increase in the rate of breathing until it ends in a gasp and a gradual decrease until the respiration stops and begins again
appliance	any device used in the mouth for functional or therapeutic effect
apprehension	uneasy anticipation
arch	collectively the teeth and bone of either the maxilla or mandible
arch forming plier	instrument used to bend or hold archwires
archwire	wire that applies pressure or force to move the teeth or to hold them in a desired position
armamentarium	anything and everything (instruments, materials, equipment, etc.) needed to complete any procedure
artery	blood vessel through which blood flows away from the heart
arteriosclerosis	pathological condition that affects the elasticity of blood vessels; "hardening of the arteries"
arthritis	inflammation of a joint(s) accompanied by pain, swelling, and stiffness
arthrogram	an x-ray of a joint (such as the TMJ) usually requiring the injection of a contrast compound into the joint capsule
arthroscope	an instrument used when viewing the inside of a joint; i.e., TMJ
articulate	to fit together; to occulate
articulating paper	paper used to register occlusal interferences
articulation	relationship between the mandible and maxilla in association with centric occlusion

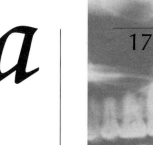

articulator	device to which mandibular and maxillary casts can be attached to maintain occlusion while reproducing movements of the temporomandibular joints
artificial ventilation (respiration)	to force oxygen into the lungs by artificial means when breathing has ceased
aseptic technique	protocol followed to minimize the chance of introducing infection or disease
aspiration	breathing in to draw foreign matter into the nose, throat, or lungs
aspirator	instrument used with a vacuum system to remove saliva and debris from the oral cavity
aspirin	an analgesic drug
assignment of benefits	authorization for the insurance company (carrier) to send payment to the dentist instead of the insured
asthma	sudden or periodic episode of wheezing and difficulty with breathing resulting from bronchospasms
astringent	agent that has a binding effect on mucous membranes and hardens tissues; an agent applied topically to control moderate bleeding by causing capillaries to constrict
asymmetry	unevenness; a lack of balance in a shape
atomize	to reduce particles into a spray
atrophy	progressive disease resulting from a decrease in cell size, number of cells, or both; often used in conjunction with muscle wasting
atropine	premedication for inhalation anesthesia used to avoid involuntary muscle spasms
attending dentist statement	dental claim form used to list the procedures performed and fees charged
attrition	gradual reduction in a material resulting from rubbing away or wearing down
augmented	to make greater; more numerous; larger or more intense
autoclave	equipment used to sterilize instruments by steam under pressure
autoclave tape	chemically treated, striped tape that changes color to provide immediate identification of processed vs. unprocessed items; does not guarantee sterilization has been achieved; used with steam sterilization

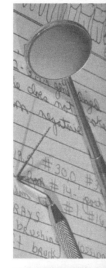

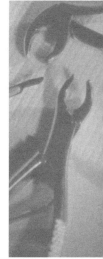

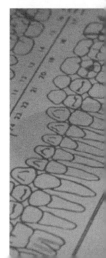

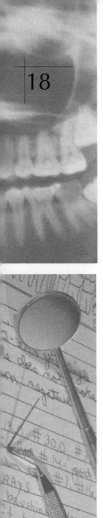

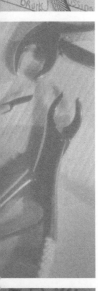

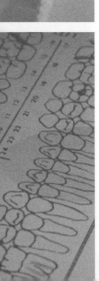

a

autogenous bone	bone taken from a part of a person's body and implanted into another part of the same person
automatic film processor	mechanical device that transports film through developing and fixing solutions along with a water wash
autopolymerization	see curing/chemical
auxiliary	any person who provides aid and assistance to a professional in the process of completing his or her work; dental assistant or hygienist
avulsed	tooth knocked out of socket
axial wall	wall of a preparation that is parallel to the long axis of the tooth

b

bacillus subtilis	generally nonpathogenic bacteria; believed to cause conjunctivitis
back up copy	a duplicate copy of stored electronic files
bacteria	one-celled plant-like microorganisms which may cause disease
bacterial biofilm	microbial species live in communities of attached bacteria in biofilm, but they also discharge free-floating single cell bacteria; biofilm bacteria are significantly more resistant to antimicrobial agents than the dispersed single cell bacteria of the same species; see biofilm
bactericidal (or bacteriocidal)	has characteristics required to destroy/kill bacteria
band driver	instrument used to push orthodontic bands into place
band pusher	instrument used in seating orthodontic molar bands for fixed appliances
band removing pliers	instrument used to remove orthodontic bands from posterior teeth
band seater	instrument used to seat orthodontic posterior metal bands onto teeth
banding	cementing of orthodontic bands to the teeth
barbed broach	endodontic instrument with protruding barbs used for the removal of the intact pulp from the canal
barriers	material used to cover dental chairs, lights, x-ray tube heads, air/water syringe, evacuators, etc. to protect against cross contamination

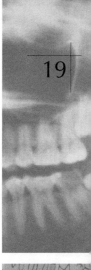

base	material placed between the cavity preparation and restorative material to protect the pulp from chemical, electrical, mechanical, or thermal irritation; not acidic; having a pH less than 7 (alkaline)
baseplate	preformed semi-ridge acrylic resin material used as a temporary denture base during the fabrication of a denture
BBP	see bloodborne pathogens
beam diameter	circumference of radiation beam; federal regulations dictate that the beam measure no more than 2.75 inches in diameter for patient and operator protection against excessive exposure to ionizing radiation
Begg appliance	a fixed orthodontic appliance modified with a ribbon-arch attachment
Bell's palsy	typically temporary facial muscle paralysis of sudden onset resulting from trauma, compression; usually serious infection of the facial nerve and identified by a distorted facial expression; recovery occurs usually without any treatment or interventions
Benadryl®	see diphenhydramine
beneficial	helpful; promoting a favorable result
benign	harmless; of no danger to one's health; non-malignant; slow growing cells that do not metastasize
Betadine®	see povidone iodine
bevel	slanted edge on the working end of an instrument; forms the cutting edge
BI	see biological indicator
biangle	instrument that has a shank with two angles; also referred to as binangle
bicuspid	see premolar
bifurcated	division of a root into two parts
binding	joining together
bioaerosols	airborne mist created from the mouth that contains microbes such as bacteria, virus, mold, fungi, and yeasts
bioburden	visible organic debris, usually blood or saliva
biofilm	a complex group of self-sufficient bacteria living together that adhere to a surface; is resistant to traditional antibiotics; in nature, biofilm is the main method of bacterial growth

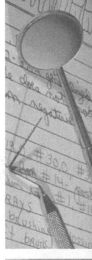

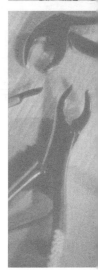

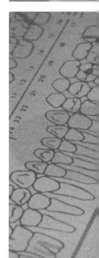

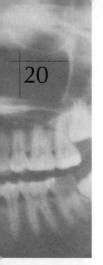

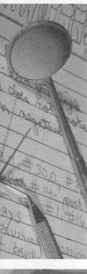

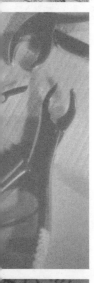

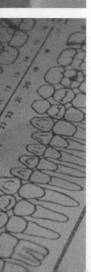

b

biological indicator (BI)	method for monitoring the sterilization process; because these indicators assess the process directly by killing known highly resistant microorganisms rather than merely testing the physical and chemical conditions necessary for sterilization; i.e., spore test
biological monitoring	process by which correct functioning of sterilization cycles are verified for each sterilizer at least weekly using biological indicators (BIs); manufacturer's directions should determine the placement and location of BI in the sterilizer; a control BI, from the same lot as the test indicator and not processed through the sterilizer, should be incubated with the test BI; the control BI should yield positive results for bacterial growth (also see spore testing)
bionator appliance	orthodontic appliance that maintains the molar position while developing the lower arch forward; see functional appliance
biopsy	tissue specimen removed from the body to distinguish malignancies from other nonmalignant lesions

Types
incisional– when a pie-shaped wedge of the suspected lesion along with normal tissue is removed

excisional– when the entire lesion is removed

bird beak pliers	instrument used to form or round an archwire and to form springs
birthday rule	regulation that stipulates the primary carrier for dependent children is determined by the parents' dates of birth, if each parent has dental coverage
bisecting angle technique	radiographic technique whereby the central x-ray is directed at an imaginary line that bisects the angle created by the long axis of the tooth and the film packet; may result in vertical distortion
bite block	plastic block with a groove for the insertion of radiograph film that is placed between the mandibular and maxillary teeth during exposure
BIS-GMA	bisphenol A diglycidylether methacrylate; foundation of synthetic resin material
biteplane	removable appliance that covers the occlusal surfaces of the mandibular or maxillary teeth to prevent articulation, generally for TMJ/TMD problems

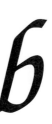

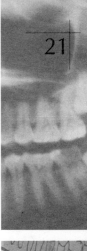

bite registration	1) measurement that shows the occlusal relationship of the maxilla and mandible for measurement of jaw relationships; 2) process that shows the occlusal relationship of the maxilla and mandible for establishment of jaw relationships; 3) a recording of desired jaw relationships that are used to transfer casts/models having the same relationship to an articulating device
bite registration materials	material used to duplicate the way the maxillary and mandibular teeth occlude
bite rim	layers of baseplate wax attached to a baseplate to reproduce the space created by missing teeth in normal occlusion; registers the vertical dimension for the denture and establishes the occlusal relationship of the mandibular and maxillary arches
bite stick	instrument with a serrated steel area used to help seat orthodontic posterior bands
bitewing radiograph	x-ray that records the coronal portion of the maxillary and mandibular teeth to diagnosis interproximal decay, evaluate restorations, detect calculus, assess the alveolar crest of bone, and tooth eruption
blanching	temporary condition characterized by a lightening in color (whitening) of the gingiva from a reduction of blood supply
bleach	see sodium hypochlorite
bleaching	cosmetic procedure performed to whiten teeth with carbamide peroxide or diluted hydrogen peroxide; internal or non-vital bleaching is performed on endodontically treated teeth with sodium perborate
block injection	see injection
Bloodborne Pathogens Standard (BBP)	federal standard created by the Occupational Health and Safety Administration (OSHA) to reduce the occupational related cases of infection, including transmission of HIV and hepatitis B, among many other infections (For a copy of the standard, go to www.osha.gov.)
blood clot	coagulation of blood into a semi-solidified state
blood glucose test	test performed to determine the sugar level of the blood
blood pressure	pressure placed by the blood upon the walls of any vessel
blurred image	radiograph that is out of focus
Board of Dental Examiners	see Board of Dentistry

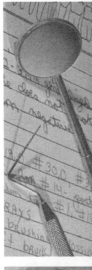

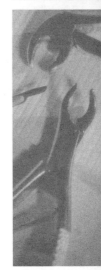

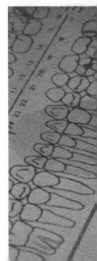

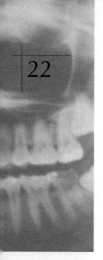
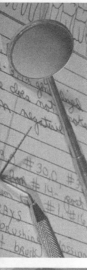
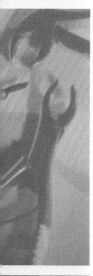
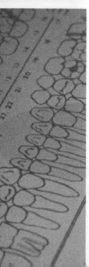

b

Board of Dentistry	state agency whose role is to define and implement regulations to guide oral healthcare professionals (often encompassing dentistry, dental hygiene, dental assisting and dental laboratory technology), in order to protect the public; also known as Board of Dental Examiners in some states
BOD	see Board of Dentistry
Boley gauge	a vernier (metric) type of measuring device accurate to tenths of millimeters
bond failure	failure of the bonding agent and filling material to adhere to the tooth surface
bonding	joining of two substances; i.e. enamel and composite material
bonding agent	material used to bond restorative materials to tooth surfaces
bone graft	transplant performed to restore bone lost as a result of periodontal disease
bone loss	destruction of bone caused by periodontal disease, tooth loss or trauma from removable prosthetics
bone substitute	synthetic osseous grafting material; often in freeze-dried form
bony impaction	unerupted tooth covered partially or completely by bone
border molding	impression compound or other material placed along the borders of a custom tray to define the length of the periphery and tissues during final denture impressions
brachial artery	main artery in the arm; used when obtaining blood pressure
brachial pulse	pulse felt in the main artery on the inside of the arm
bracket	attachment welded to orthodontic bands or bonded directly to teeth to hold an archwire
bracket forceps	hinged instrument used to hold orthodontic brackets for placement and positioning
bracket placement tweezers	instrument used to place orthodontic brackets on the facial surface of a tooth
bracket slots	horizontal slots in an orthodontic bracket into which the archwire fits
bradycardia	slowing of the pulse rate along with an abnormal slowness of the heart (pulse rate under 50 beats per minute)

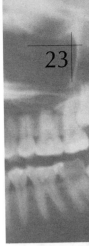

bradypnea	abnormally slow respiration rate when at rest
breach of contract	act of not abiding to the arrangements in a written document or verbal agreement
Bremsstahlung radiation	refers to the sudden stopping (deceleration) of electrons as they interact with positively charged nuclei; referred to as braking radiation
Brevital®	see methohexital sodium
bridge	prosthesis permanently cemented that replaces one or more teeth
brass wire	separator that is placed between the contacts of teeth forcing them apart to make space for an orthodontic band
broach	fine instrument used in Endodontic procedures to locate and remove the contents (pulp) of the root canal

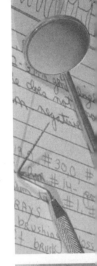

Types
barbed–	surface covered with small barbs, points or spikes, used to extirpate (grab and pull out) pulp tissues
smooth–	without barbs; used for exploring fine and tortuous (full of turns and twists) root canals

broad spectrum	antibiotic with wide range effectiveness against bacterial infection
brochospasms	spasms of the bronchus; involuntary contraction of the bronchioles, leading to wheezing; may result in an asthma attack
bronchi	two large branches leading from the trachea that are the passageway for air going to and from the lungs (bronchus = one bronchi)
bronchial asthma	see asthma

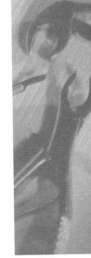

bronchitis	inflammation of the bronchial mucous membrane characterized by coughing, fever, rapid pulse, soreness behind the sternum, and dyspnea on exertion
bronchospasms	spasm of the bronchus; involuntary contraction of the bronchioles, leading to wheezing; may result in an asthma attack
bruise	see ecchymosis; see hematoma
bruxism	involuntary gnashing, grinding, or clenching of teeth
buccal	surface adjacent to the cheek

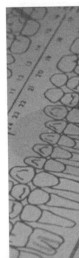

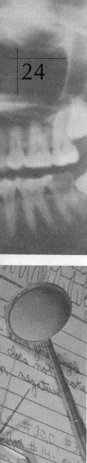
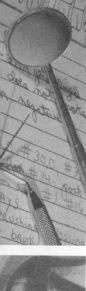
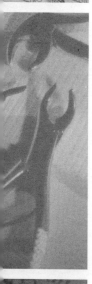
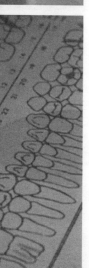

24

b

buccal nerve branch	nerves that pass through the buccinator muscle to the cheek where it enters into the buccal mucosa, buccal gingiva, and the buccal of the mandibular molars
buccal tube	small cylindrical tube located on the buccal portion of an orthodontic molar band that serves as an attachment for the labial archwire
buccal vestibule	space located between the alveolar ridge and teeth, and the cheek
buccinator	muscle of facial expression; compresses the cheek and retracts the angle of the mouth
buffer period	time in a schedule for emergencies or for completion of tasks that need to be completed
bulbous	rounded or swollen
bulimia	an eating disorder characterized by vomiting of food resulting in erosion of the lingual surfaces of the maxillary incisors
bulk quantity orders	ordering of supplies in a large quantity, typically for products that do not have a shelf life
bur	see rotary cutting instruments
Burlew® wheel	abrasive, knife edged, rubber polishing wheel used to smooth metallic restorations and tooth surfaces
burnish	to make smooth or glossy by rubbing or polishing
BWX	see bitewing radiographs (x-rays)

C

calcification	1) deposition of calcium salts and other materials when teeth are developing; 2) when plaque absorbs mineral salts found in saliva and converted into calculus
calcify	harden
calcium	nutrient needed for mineralization of bone and teeth
calcium hydroxide	material used for pulp capping for its therapeutic effect on the pulp; promotes formation of secondary dentin and can be used as a cavity liner
calculus	mineralized plaque that becomes hard and rough when calcium salts and other minerals are deposited into plaque; forms on teeth, restorations, and removable appliances

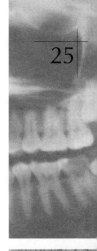

Caldwell-Luc procedure	operation to remove disease or chronically inflammed mucosa in the maxillary sinus through an opening through the front of the sinus, under the lip above the gingiva of the upper teeth an artificial drainage pathway is created between the sinus and the nasal passage
camosurface	junction of the wall of the cavity
candidiasis	fungal pathology caused by Candida albicans and characterized by white fungal patches that scrape off and leave bleeding bases; commonly called thrush
canine	tooth with just one cusp; located between the lateral incisors and first premolars in each quadrant; purpose is to tear food; has one root and one root canal; see root canal
canker sore	circular painful lesion with a yellowish center and red ring around the lesion; associated with heredity, trauma, stress, food allergens and hormonal changes; also called aphthous stomatitis (aphthous ulcer)
canthus	refers to either corner (outer or inner) of the eye; often used in dental radiology to help in placing the position indicating device (PID) for maxillary canine (cuspid) exposures
capital expenditures	money spent to purchase or upgrade major equipment or for office improvements
capitation dental insurance plan	plan that pays a fixed fee on a monthly basis to provide care to patients assigned to the practice, whether service is rendered or not; (after the fixed fee has been paid, no additional payment is made to the practice for any services rendered)
carbamide peroxide	agent used to whiten teeth
cardiac	pertaining to the heart
cardiac arrest	condition where the heart beat ceases or the heart fails to function
cardiac arrhythmia	change in force, quality and sequence of normal heart rhythm
cardiac dysrythmia	disordered heart rhythm
cardiopulmonary resuscitation (CPR)	life saving procedure that combines artificial respiration with external cardiac massage

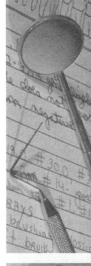

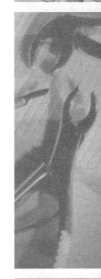

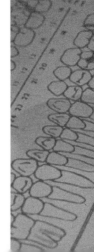

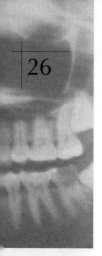
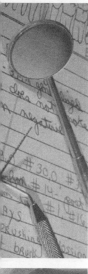
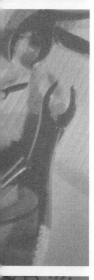
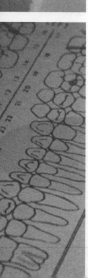

C

caries	tooth decay

Types
arrested– decay showing no progression

incipient– beginning decay

rampant– widespread or growing decay

recurrent– decay under or near margins of restorations

cariogenic caries (cavity) production or generation

carotid artery main artery located on each side of the neck that carries the principal blood supply to the head and neck

carotid pulse expansion and contraction of the carotid artery caused by surges of the blood flow in concert with the heart beat

Carpule® (cartridge) glass cylinder container with a pre-measured amount of sterile anesthetic solution

carrier person who carries a disease often without obvious symptoms and is capable of transmitting disease with or without contact with another person

cartilage dense, flexible connective tissue; located on the joint surfaces of some bones

carver instrument with a carving (less sharp) edge rather than a cutting (sharp) edge used to shape restorative materials

cassette metal or vinyl holder used to hold extraoral radiographic film

catalyst substance used to initiate the setting reaction of a material

cathode portion of the x-ray tube that produces a negative charge and supplies the electrons necessary to produce x-rays

caustic property of a substance that is capable of burning or corroding

cauterize to burn tissue; apart/separate through the use of electricity

cavity classifications classification of cavities according to the surfaces of a tooth in which decay is present; initially developed by Dr. G.V. Black in the late 1800's

Class I– decay found in pits and fissures on the occlusal 2/3 of posterior teeth or the lingual surface on anterior teeth

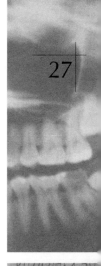

cavity classifications *(continued)*	Class II–	decay on proximal surfaces of premolars and molars
	Class III–	decay on proximal surfaces of anterior teeth (canines and incisors)
	Class IV–	decay on proximal surfaces of anterior teeth (canines and incisors) that involves the incisal angle
	Class V–	decay in the gingival third of a tooth that involves the facial (labial, buccal) or lingual (palatal) surfaces
	Class VI–	decay on the incisal edges and cusps of teeth

cavity preparation removal of decay and shaping of tooth structure done in order for the tooth to receive restorative materials

Types
simple– involving one surface

compound– involving two surfaces

complex– involving three or more surfaces

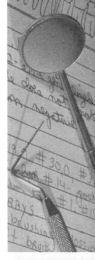

cavity varnish agent used to seal dentinal tubules to prevent acids, saliva and debris from reaching the pulp

cavosurface junction of the wall of the cavity

CDC see Centers for Disease Control and Prevention; see listing in Appendix A

CEJ see cementoenamel junction

celluloid crown form clear plastic form that can be filled with acrylic to fabricate a provisional restoration

cement material that produces a mechanical bond between two surfaces; relatively low-strength materials used when strength is not a major consideration; few cements form adhesive bonds with enamel or dentin but they possess many desirable characteristics

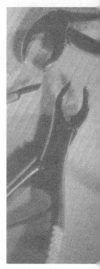

cementoblasts cells that form the cementum

cementoenamel junction (CEJ) point where the cementum and enamel meet

cementum thin layer of modified bone formed by cementoblasts deposited on the dentin of the root of the tooth to which the periodontal ligament attaches

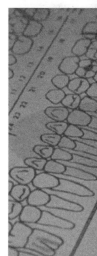

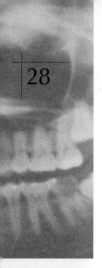

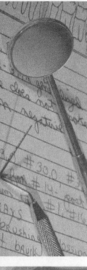

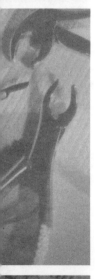

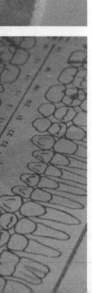

C

Centers for Disease Control and Prevention (CDC)
an independent agency that investigates, reports and tracks specific diseases; a nationally recognized agency regarding issues concerning public health

central beam
see central ray

central incisor
tooth located on either side of the midline on both arches with the primary purpose of cutting food; there are four central incisors in the permanent and four central incisors in the primary dentitions; has one root canal

central ray
primary ray or beam emitted from the x-ray tubehead that consists of hard x-rays with short wavelengths

centric occlusion
occlusion that occurs when the condyle rests in the temporal bone while biting in an unstrained position on the posterior teeth

cephalometric radiograph
extraoral radiograph of the head that is used in orthodontic and prosthodontic dentistry to show a profile of the patient's head

cephalometric tracing
lines or patterns drawn of structures from a cephalometric radiograph made on translucent film to evaluate relationships among anatomical landmarks

cerebral function
brain activity

Certified Dental Assistant (CDA®)
dental assistant who has successfully challenged the national DANB Certification exam consisting of three component exams: the General Chairside assisting (GC) exam, the Radiation Health & Safety (RHS) exam and the Infection Control (ICE) exam; the CDA exam is administered by the Dental Assisting National Board, Inc. (DANB); the CDA requires annual renewal

Certified Dental Practice Management Administrator (CDPMA®)
dental assistant who has successfully challenged the national DANB Certification exam in Dental Practice Management Administration (CDPMA); the CDPMA exam is administered by the Dental Assisting National Board, Inc. (DANB); the CDPMA requires annual renewal

Certified Dental Technician
laboratory technician who has successfully challenged an examination in dental laboratory skills administered by the National Board for Certification

Certified Oral and Maxillofacial Surgery Assistant (COMSA®)
dental assistant who has successfully challenged the national DANB Certification exam consisting of two component exams: the Oral and Maxillofacial Surgery (OMSA) Assisting exam and the Infection Control (ICE) exam; the COMSA exam was administered by the Dental Assisting National Board, Inc. (DANB) before 2000; the COMSA requires annual renewal

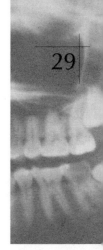

C

Certified Orthodontic Assistant (COA®)	dental assistant who has successfully challenged the national DANB certification exam consisting of two component exams: the Orthodontic Assisting (OA) exam and the Infection Control (ICE) exam ; the COA exam is administered by the Dental Assisting National Board, Inc. (DANB); the COA requires annual renewal
cervical	pertaining to neck; such as neck of the tooth
cervical abrasion	abnormal wearing away of the cervical portion of a tooth or teeth, caused by improper tooth brushing or flossing technique
cervical (thyroid) collar	used in addition to a lead apron to reduce exposure to the neck area
cervical margin	junction that divides the anatomical crown from the root of the tooth
cfu/ml	acronym for colony-forming units per milliliter of water
chalk	mild abrasive used in some prophylactic pastes; inert filler used in many dental materials
chamfer	in crown preparations, a marginal finish that produces a curve from the axial wall to the cavosurface; see cavosurface
charge slip	form that acts as an invoice and a receipt for the patient with the surface of the tooth
cheek retractor	instrument used to pull back or retract the cheek during invasive procedures or intraoral photography
cheilosis	a non-inflammatory condition of the lip usually characterized by chapping and fissuring (cracking the corners of the mouth)
chelation	chemical reaction of a metallic ion with a reactive compound to form a compound in which the metal ion is tightly bound
chemical bond	the force that holds two or more units of matter together by a change in the structure of the matter
chemical burn	burn to tissues caused by caustic materials
chemical cure	see curing
chemical disinfectant	liquid used for disinfection of hard surfaces and instruments

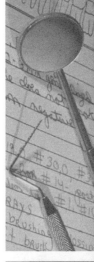

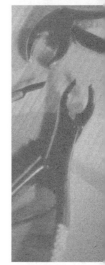

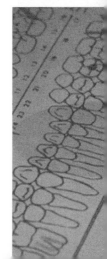

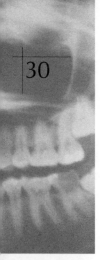
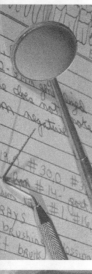
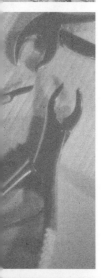
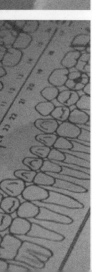

C

chemical indicator	use of sensitive chemicals to assess physical conditions (i.e., time and temperature) during the sterilization process; they do not prove sterilization but they allow detection of certain equipment malfunctions and they help to identify procedural errors

Types

external indicator–	applied to the outside packaging (i.e., chemical indicator tape or special marks) change color rapidly when a specific parameter (temperature) is reached and verify that the package has been exposed to the sterilization process
internal indicator–	used inside each package to ensure the sterilizing agent has penetrated the packaging material and actually reached the instruments inside

chemical labeling	diamond-shaped label with four colors: blue, yellow, red, and white, that is placed on a container with numbers and codes to identify a specific hazard category
chemical retention	joining of restorative materials to a cavity preparation or tooth surface through chemical reaction
chemical vapor sterilization	process that sterilizes using an unsaturated chemical vapor (a combination of pressure and chemicals); see chemiclave
chemiclave	unsaturated chemical vapor unit used to sterilize instruments through chemical vapor sterilization
chemotherapy	administration of chemical agents that have a toxic effect on a disease-causing microorganism
chisel	an instrument (single- or double-ended) with a single bevel (straight or angles) cutting edge used to cleave (cut) or plane (smooth) both enamel and dentin walls of a cavity preparation
chlorhexidine	medicament used to treat gingivitis; reduces the inflammation, swelling, and bleeding of gingiva
chlorhexidine gluconate	germicide used to reduce bacteria in the mouth and in hand wash
chrome cobalt	metal alloy used for the framework of partial dentures and for metallic denture bases
chronic	lasting for a long period of time or marked by frequent occurrence; frequently symptoms are less severe but last for a longer period of time
chronic exposure	long term, frequent exposure to a damaging entity

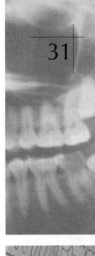

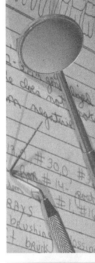

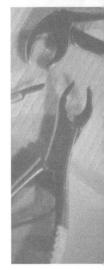

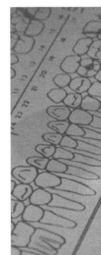

chronological age	age from time of occurrence or birth; actual age
chuck	metal cylinder in the head of a handpiece or on a bench (polishing) lathe that holds a bur or mandrel
cingulum	convex band of enamel on the lingual surface of anterior teeth near the gingival margin
circulating assistant	dental assistant that assists the primary chairside assistant
circumference	area around a closed circular space; perimeter of a circle
circumvallate	to surround; surrounded by a trough or ridge; to be under
circumvallate papillae (or vallate papillae)	see papillae
claimant	person who files a claim for benefits; the patient or subscriber
claim form	form that lists the date and service performed along with the fees charged; submitted to insurance carrier for payment
classifications of motion	movements employed during instrument transfer and during instrumentation

	Class I–	finger movement only
	Class II–	finger and wrist movement
	Class III–	finger, wrist and elbow movement
	Class IV–	arm and shoulder movement
	Class V–	arm movement and twisting of the body

clasp	device that holds a removable appliance in the mouth
clean	removal of debris/bioburden to give the subsequent sterilization or disinfection step the best chance to work
clear film	radiographic film that has not been exposed to radiation or has been subject to processing errors such as being left in the fixer or wash for a prolonged period of time, resulting in a lack of evidence of exposure
cleat(s)	fixed anchor in the form of a metal spur or loop embedded into the base of a Hawley retainer or soldered onto an archwire to which an elastic or other mechanism is attached
cleave	to cut, split or separate

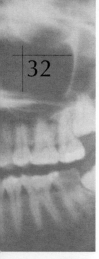

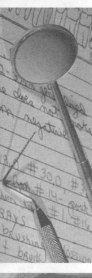

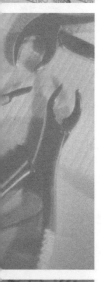

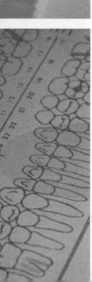

32

C

cleft lip	congenital separation of the upper lip caused by failure of the maxillary process to fuse with the medial nasal process
cleft palate	congenital fissure in the roof of the mouth resulting from an incomplete fusion of the palate during development
clinical contact surfaces	those surfaces that can be directly contaminated from patient materials either by direct spray or spatter generated during dental procedures or by contact with DHCP's gloved hands; these surfaces (i.e., light handles, switches, drawer handles, pens, etc.) can subsequently contaminate other instruments, devices, hands, or gloves
clinical crown	portion of the tooth covered by enamel and that is visible in the mouth; usually a portion of the enamel is covered by gingival, but if recession has occurred, the clinical crown and the anatomical crown can become the same thing
clinical examination	visual inspection of the tissues in and surrounding the oral cavity
clinical record	collection of all information regarding a patient's treatment that includes, but is not limited to: diagnosis, observations, completed procedures, fees charged and payments received
CNS	acronym for central nervous system
coagulation	process of clotting
coalesce	to fuse together
coin test	test performed to see if there are white light leaks in the darkroom or daylight loader; part of quality assurance process
cold pack	packet containing a coolant used after oral surgery to control swelling
collection agency	organization retained to collect on past due accounts
college pliers	see cotton pliers
collimator	lead plate with a hole in the middle that restricts the size of an x-ray beam; increased safety of exposure to ionizing radiation
comatose	unconscious
commissure	corner of the mouth
communicable disease	disease that may be transmitted directly or indirectly from one individual to another
Compazine®	see prochlorperazine

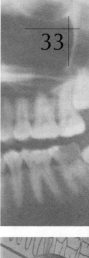

composite	resin restorative material that is hardened by chemical or light curing
Comprehensive Drug Abuse Prevention and Control Act of 1970	federal act established to identify drugs according to five schedules of abuse potential; Title II of this act deals with the control and enforcement of drugs
compress	to press together into a smaller mass
compressed gas cylinders	containers that hold gases, i.e., oxygen, nitrous oxide
compule	single-application cartridge of bonding or restorative material
concave	surface that curves inward
condensation	1) gas or vapor that changes into a liquid 2) compressing of restorative materials
condense	compressing material into a cavity preparation
conducting agent	substance, such as tooth paste, that will transmit an electrical impulse
condyle	rounded process (projection of bone; elevation) at the end of the ramus of the mandible that fits into the glenoid fossa and is a component of the temporomandibular joint
cone cut	radiographic exposure error created by incorrect alignment of the central x-ray beam resulting in a non-exposed portion on the film
conference call	call where more than two people can talk from various locations on the telephone at the same time
congenital	present at birth
congestive heart failure	disease state caused by retention of sodium and fluids due to cardiac or kidney disorders resulting in the heart being unable to reach the level of cardiac output the body needs
conical	cone shaped
conjunctivitis	infection resulting in inflammation of the mucous membrane that lines the eyelids
connective tissue graft	procedure performed to treat root exposures; a flap of tissue is cut from the roof of the mouth, the underlying tissue is removed, the flap is sutured back to the roof of the mouth; the removed tissue is slipped under the gum tissue surrounding an exposed root surface and anchored in place with sutures
conscious sedation	patient is sedated to pain or anxiety, but retains the ability to respond to simple commands

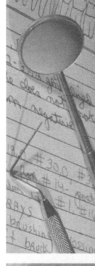

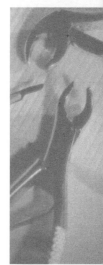

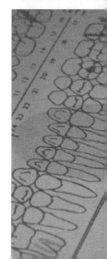

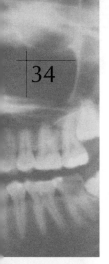
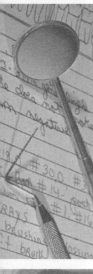
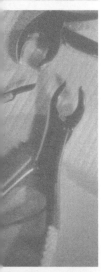
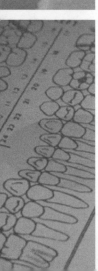

C

consent	permission

<u>Types</u>

implied– when the patient freely opens his or her mouth for the dentist to begin treatment

informed– written agreement by the patient allowing the dentist to perform procedures after being informed of what procedures need to be done, risks involved, alternate treatment options, and expected outcome

consent waiver form signed by a patient or guardian granting permission to perform a specified procedure

consultation
1) meeting between the dentist and patient (parent, guardian, and/or person responsible for payment) to discuss the diagnosis and to present a treatment plan
2) meeting between the patient and another dental or medical professional for the purpose of advancing the patient's dental care beyond that of the referring dentist

contact dermatitis an inflammation of the skin as a result of direct contact with a microorganism

contact points area on the proximal surface of adjacent teeth where the two teeth touch

contamination introducing any surface, instrument, or person to a non-sterile, often infectious agent

contiguous something that is adjacent to or touching

continuous simple suture suture that does not end except at the beginning and end of an incision; used in cases of multiple extractions

continuous sling suture series of surgical sutures used where a large flap has been laid involving multiple teeth and both facial and lingual surfaces

contour
1) to manipulate into a desired shape contour
2) outline or external shape of a surface

contouring pliers instrument used to contour bands into shape to adapt to a tooth

contra angle see handpiece

contract binding agreement between two or more competent parties of consenting age obligating each party to do or not to do a specific thing; agreement between two or more competent parties in which an offer is made and accepted and each party benefits; can be formal, informal, written, oral or just plain understood; some contracts are required to be in writing in order to be enforced

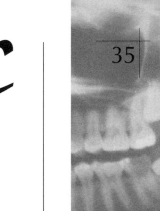

contraindicated	symptom or condition that indicates a possible reaction other than what is desired or proper
contrast	differences in the degree of blackness between various structures on a radiograph
convex	surface that bulges outward
convulsions	intense, involuntary muscular contraction; seizures
Coons ligature pliers	instrument used to manipulate ligature wire
copayment	amount of the total approved amount that the subscriber is obligated to pay
COPD	acronym for chronic obstructive pulmonary disease
coping	like a cap or covering of thin metal over a prepared tooth
coronal	pertaining to the crown portion of the tooth
coronal polish	polishing of the clinical crown of a tooth
coronoid process	point of insertion for the fiber bundles of the temporal muscle; the front tip of the ramus
corpuscle	any small body, mass, or organ, such as a blood cell or an encapsulated sensory nerve ending
corrode	to rust
corrosion	surface disintegration resulting from prolonged chemical or electrochemical contact
cortical plate (bone)	dense compact bone that makes up part of the alveolar process
cotton forceps	see cotton pliers
cotton pellet	ball of cotton used to place medicaments, solutions or to dry
cotton pledget	see cotton pellet
cotton pliers	instrument used to carry small objects to and from the oral cavity
cotton rolls	absorbent rolls of cotton material used to control moisture and for the isolation of teeth
Coumadin®	an oral anticoagulant (blood thinner) generically known as warfarin sodium; see warfarin sodium
CPR	see cardiopulmonary resuscitation

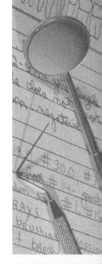

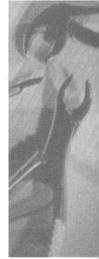

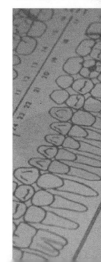

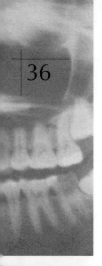

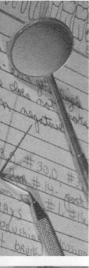

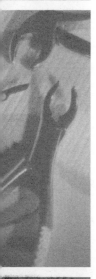

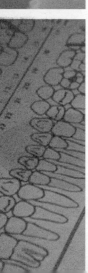

C

Crabtree	a device used in dental radiography for normalizing and monitoring the quality of radiograph processing solutions as part of a quality control program; used for measuring proper film density from processing solutions
cratered	pitted; concave
CRE	acronym for central ray entry; see central ray
crepitus	a crackling sound as that produced by the rubbing together of a fractured bone or by air moving in a tissue space (crepitation)
criminal law	deals with cases involving crimes committed against society, including fraud, practicing dentistry without a license, and inappropriate use of drugs, and crimes committed against another person, including abuse of patients
crimp	to bend or mold into a desired shape or to pinch together
Crohn's disease	a chronic inflammatory disease of the intestines which primarily causes ulcerations in the small and large intestines, but can affect the digestive system anywhere between the mouth and the anus; the disease is found in equal frequency in men and women, and usually is first diagnosed in patients in their teens or early twenties
crossbite	line of occlusion where the mandibular teeth are anterior and/or buccal to the maxillary teeth
cross-contamination	transferring non-sterile, often infectious agents from one surface, instrument or patient to another
cross-sectional exposure	exposure of an occlusal radiograph where the central x-ray is perpendicular to the film
crown	reproduction of a clinical crown made of gold alloys, porcelain, stainless steel ,combination of gold fused to porcelain, or other materials
Crozat appliance	removable orthodontic appliance used to widen the maxillary and mandibular arches
CT	acronym for computerized tomography
culture	to attempt to grow microorganisms in an artificial medium
culturing	controlled processes for growing microorganisms or other living cells on artificial media (different forms of agar)
cumulative effects	increasing level of effect
cumulative exposure	total accumulated exposure resulting from repeated radiation exposures

curettage	removal of diseased periapical tissue, debridement and planing to smooth the surfaces of the roots and removal of calculus by use of a curette
curette **(or curete)**	periodontal or surgical instrument used for debridement and for root and gingival curettage
curing	hardening of material by chemical reaction or light exposure

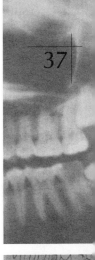

Types

chemical **or self–**	mixing of a base and catalyst together to create a chemical reaction resulting in the hardening of a material (autopolymerization)
light–	process employed to cure (set) a photo-sensitive material
dual–	some hardening takes place as the material is mixed; the final hardening does not take place until the material is exposed to a light source

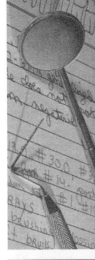

curing light	high-density, visible light that cures (sets or hardens) photo-sensitive materials; i.e., composite
cusp	pointed or rounded protrusion on the coronal portion of a tooth
cuspid	see canine
cuspidor	bowl with flowing, circulating water into which the patients expectorates (spits)
Cusp of Carabelli	fifth cusp located on the mesiolingual surface of most maxillary first molars

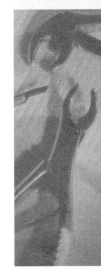

cutting edge	sharp edge of an instrument formed by a straight surface and a beveled surface meeting at less than a 45° angle; used in a restoration preparation
cyanoacrylate	glue that bonds instantly upon application
cyanotic	patient presents with a bluish, grayish discoloration of the skin caused by poorly oxygenated blood
cyclopropane	flammable colorless gas used as an anesthetic
cytologic smear	bacteria taken from an area or lesion that is placed on a slide for microscopic examination

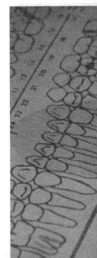

cyst	space in bone or tissue which contains a fluid or semifluid material

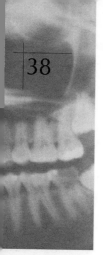

d

dappen dish	small glass, metal or rubber container used to hold solutions, pumice, prophylaxis paste, etc.
darkroom	light proof room used to process radiographs
dark spots	radiographic processing error caused by developer being splashed on exposed film before processing
daysheet	listing of activities for patients that includes, but is not limited to: procedures performed, fees charged, payments received, and balances for a specific day
DDS	Doctor of Dental Surgery
deactivate	to render ineffective
debride	removal of plaque and calculus from teeth supragingivally and subgingivally; to remove debris from a root canal or to remove dead tissue
debris	accumulation of excess or foreign material attached to a surface
Decadron®	see dexamethasone
decalcification	beginning of decay (caries) on the outside surface of a tooth in either the enamel or cementum through the loss of calcium salts from calcified tissues such as enamel
decay	see caries
decontamination	to remove infectious agents from surfaces or instruments
deductible	dollar amount the patient must pay toward the cost of treatment before an insurance company begins to pay benefits for treatment received
defamation of character	act of causing injury to a person's reputation, name, or character verbally or in writing
dehydration	decrease of fluids in the body
delegate	to appoint someone to perform an act or carry out a task
Demerol®	see meperidine
demineralization	process whereby minerals, such as calcium and phosphate, are lost from the tooth or enamel; early stage of decay process
demographic information	individual identifying information that frequently includes the name, address, telephone number and birth date of a patient; considered protected health information (PHI) by the Health Insurance Portability & Accountability Act (HIPAA)

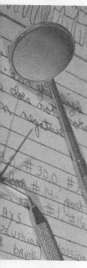

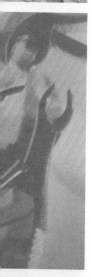

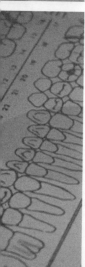

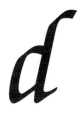

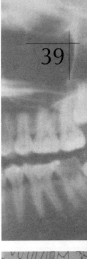

dense	difficult to penetrate; compact; allowing little or no light to penetrate; particles or atoms located close together
density	level of darkness/denseness
dental dam	thin sheet of rubber (latex) or non-latex substitute used to isolate a tooth or teeth from contamination from saliva and/or blood; frequently referred to as rubber dam
dental dam clamp (retainer)	devise made with or without wings (projections on the edges of the jaws used to help with keeping the dental (rubber) dam in place) to aid in the retention and retraction of the dental dam

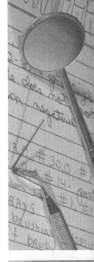

dental dam forceps	hinged instrument used to place and remove dental dam clamps (retainers)
dental dam frame	u-shaped (Young's), or circular (Ostby frame) frame work, as well as straps to hold the dam material away from the working area
dental dam napkin	fabric placed under a dental dam used to absorb fluids and to prevent the dental dam from coming into contact with the patient's skin and causing irritation
dental dam punch	instrument used to punch holes in the dental dam
dental floss	thin string-like material used to remove plaque from proximal surfaces and debris from interproximal spaces of teeth

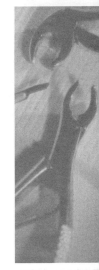

Types

ribbon/tape– flat, wide floss coated with wax; additional strength often used when food is impacted between teeth

waxed– braided filaments of material coated with wax; often used for tight or rough contacts but will leave a coating of wax on the tooth surface

unwaxed– braided filaments of material without any wax; cleans fairly well and does not leave a waxy coating on the tooth but tends to break

ultra fine– individual filaments of material that tend to flatten out when depressed against a surface; provides more surface for cleaning but tends to fray more easily

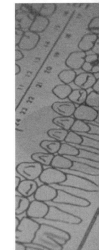

Dental Practice Act	state-specific regulations that outline the rules governing acts allowable by law that are performed by a dentist, assistant, hygienist, and laboratory technician in that particular state

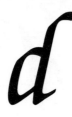

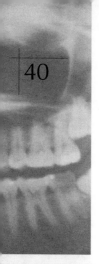

d

dental public health	science and art of preventing and controlling dental diseases and promoting dental health through organized community efforts; a form of dental practice that serves the community as a patient rather than the individual that is concerned with the dental health education of the public, with applied dental research, and with the administration of group dental care programs as well as the prevention and control of dental diseases on a community basis
dental pulp	see pulp
dentifrice	substance used to cleanse the teeth; i.e. toothpaste.
dentin	calcified tissue that forms the major part of the tooth; softer than enamel
dentin (secondary)	dentin formed on the walls of pulp chambers and canals (before the tooth is completely formed) because of disturbances that result from stimulation of the odontoblasts; can be chemically stimulated by calcium hydroxide placed on the floor of the preparation when decay is close to the pulp
dentinal tubule	tube that passes through dentin from the pulp to the dentinoenamel junction that transmits pain and nutrition
dentition	natural teeth in the maxillary and mandibular arches
denture	removable prosthesis that replaces all teeth
denture base	portion of a denture made of acrylic that holds artificial teeth
deposit	to put money into a checking or savings account at a financial institution; to place on a surface
dermatitis	inflammation of the skin that presents with itching, redness and various lesions
desensitize	to make insensitive or non-reactive to stimulation from touch or temperature
deteriorate	to disintegrate, decay or break down
detrimental	to cause damage or harm
developer	solution that brings out the latent image on an exposed radiographic film
developmental age	age related to the developmental stage of a child
developmental groove	grooves on the surfaces of teeth that separate portions of the tooth from each other

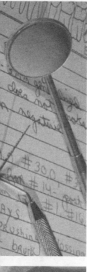

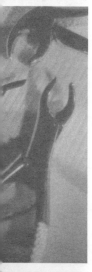

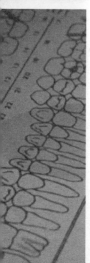

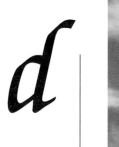

dexamethasone	anti-inflammatory drug; generic name for Decadron®
dextrose	see glucose
DHCW	acronym for dental healthcare worker
DHCP	acronym for dental healthcare personnel
diabetes mellitus	condition created from a high level of glucose in the blood because of insufficient insulin production; may lead to medical emergencies; important in patient scheduling
diabetic coma	medical emergency caused by the lack of insulin in the system; can be reversible but is life-threatening
diagnosis	determination made by the dentist from a collection of diagnostic data and information regarding a patient's condition

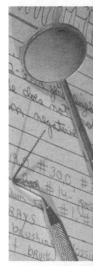

diaphragm	1) plate usually made of lead, with a small opening to limit the beam of radiation for exposing radiographs 2) a muscle wall that separates the abdomen from the thorax which expands and contracts with each inhalation to permit entry of air into the lungs
diastema	space between two teeth in the same arch
diastolic pressure	the second ending (last) sound heard while taking blood pressure; reflects the heart muscle at rest when it is allowing the heart to take in blood before the next contraction
diazepam	a Schedule IV controlled substance used in dentistry to reduce anxiety; a CNS depressant drug used to manage short-term anxiety disorders and symptoms of anxiety; may also be used for conscious sedation; generic name for Valium®

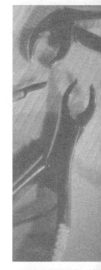

die stone	gypsum product that is used where a very strong and/or accurate model or cast is needed
diffusion	act of spreading out or scattering
digest	to convert a substance so that it can be absorbed by the body
digestible	easy to digest
digital radiography	computerized radiographic process that utilizes sensor rather than single use film and reduces exposure of radiation to a patient by 90% or more
digitalis	drug used to aid in increasing the contraction of the heart muscle, increasing the output of the heart, and a decrease in heart size; generic name for Lanoxin® (digoxin)

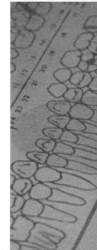

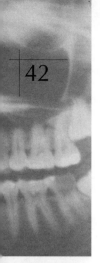
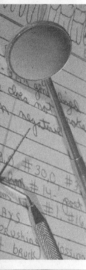
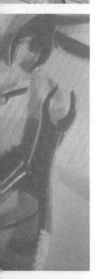
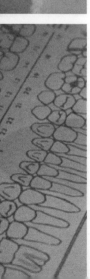

d

digoxin	see digitalis
Dilantin®	see phenytoin
dilated pupils	pupils that are larger than normal in circumference
dilute	to reduce concentration of a liquid resulting in a reduction in strength
dimensional change	change from the original size or shape of an object usually caused by temperature change or loss of water (syneresis) or absorption of water (imbibtion)
diminish	to reduce or make smaller
diphenhydramine	antihistamine used to reduce effects of an allergic reaction; generic name for Benadryl®
direct supervision	see supervision
disadvantage	to place an individual or individuals in an unfavorable condition
discard	throw away
disclosing agents	red or fluorescent yellow dye applied to the teeth to stain plaque to aid with oral hygiene instruction
discs	instruments used to polish, smooth and adjust restorative materials and appliances

<u>Types</u>

carborundum–	double sided disc used to cut and finish gold restorations
diamond disc–	steel disc used for rapid cutting with diamond particles or chips bonded to both sides of the disc
lightening–	steel separating disc used to cut metal
polishing–	has an extremely fine abrasive used to finish and polish a surface
sandpaper disc–	has abrasive material on one side of the disc and sizes: garnet, sand, emery and cuttlefish

disengage	to release or disconnect
disinfect	process of killing most pathogenic microorganisms but not bacterial endospores

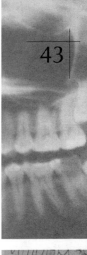

disinfectant	chemical intended for use on instruments and touch surfaces to destroy most pathogenic microorganisms
disinfection	the process of killing pathogens by physical or chemical means; it does not destroy spores and resistant viruses

Types

high-level–	destroys all disease-producing microbes but not necessarily high levels of bacterial spores
intermediate level –	destroys vegetative bacteria, most fungi and most viruses; is tuberculocidal
low-level–	destroys vegetative bacteria, some fungi and some viruses; is not tuberculocidal

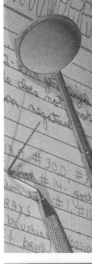

disintegrate	to break down
dislodge	to move from position by force or energy
dissipate	to lose energy or evaporate
distal	surface of the tooth away from the midline
distal end cutter	hinged instrument used to cut an archwire after it has been placed in the buccal tube
distortion	a change from original shape
distract	to take attention away from current situation
ditching	1) loss of enamel along the margin of a restoration 2) process used to make the margin of a crown preparation more obvious on a die

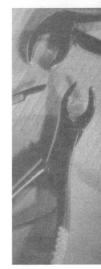

divergent	to go into different or opposite directions or to differ in any way
DMD	Doctor of Medical Dentistry
don	to put on
dorsum	upper and outer surface of an organ; top surface of the tongue
dosage	quantity of medication given to produce a desired effect
dosimeter	detection badge for monitoring exposure to radiation
double exposure	technique error where a film has been exposed to radiation twice resulting in two images showing on the film

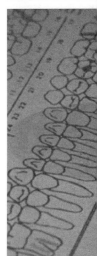

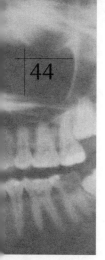
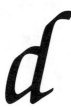

d

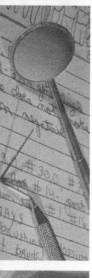

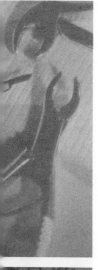

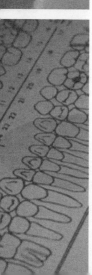

double film packet	film packet that contains two films allowing for the production of two identical radiographs
downloading	transferring information received over a communications network to a software program so that it can be accessed
Down Syndrome	congenital disorder characterized by mild mental retardation; often accompanied by short stature and flattened facial profile
down time	time in the appointment schedule that is not used to book appointments
Doxycycline®	a tetracycline use in the treatment of periodontal disease
DPA	see Dental Practice Act
DPM	acronym for Dental Practice Management
drain	channel for release or discharge from a wound
drifting	movement of a tooth or teeth into a space left empty from a missing tooth or teeth
droplet infection	produced by introduction of pathogens into the air by coughing, sneezing, or talking
drug interaction	increased or decreased effect one drug can have on another when both are taken at the same time
dry heat sterilization	method of sterilization using a convection oven
dry socket	painful condition resulting from failure of a blood clot formation or when the blood clot is washed from the extraction site, exposing the nerve endings over the bone; see alveolitis
dual cure	see curing
duplication film	film used only to duplicate processed radiographs
duplication machine	equipment that uses white light to expose/ transfer an image on already processed film on to duplication film
DUWL	acronym for dental unit waterlines
dysfunction	malfunction; not functioning correctly or at all
dyspnea	difficulty with breathing resulting in shortness of breath usually associated with lung or heart disease

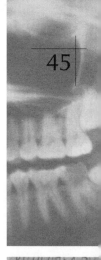

east-west Cryer elevator	surgical elevator used for the removal of root fragments or tips
ecchymosis	passage of blood from ruptured blood vessels into subcutaneous tissue marked by a purplish discoloration of the tissue; a bruise; see hemotoma
ectopic beat	cardiac heart beat beginning at a point other than the medically designated starting point
edema	swelling of any tissue or organ
edentulous	without teeth, partially or completely
edgewise appliance	orthodontic appliance with attachment brackets and a rectangular slot for a round or rectangular archwire
edgewise plier	hinged instrument used to hold or adjust archwires
effective	having a favorable influence
effective date	date an insurance plan or contract goes into effect
egress	going out; an exit
EKG	see electrocardiogram
elastic chain	chain of continuous Os that attaches to orthodontic brackets on several adjacent teeth to bring teeth together
elastics	latex circles (orthodontic rubber bands) available in a variety of sizes used to provide pulling forces for tooth movement
elastic separator	small donut-shaped plastic circles placed between the contacts of teeth forcing them apart to make space for an orthodontic band
elective	having a choice
electrocardiogram	recording of the electrical activity of the heart used to diagnose abnormal cardiac rhythms
electrocauterization/electrosurgery	surgical process of cutting tissues while coagulating the blood at the same time by means of a wire embedded in a holder that is heated by electricity
elevator	instrument used to free gingiva from the underlying bone as well as to loosen and/or remove teeth, root tips, and root fragments; there are several shapes and designs
eligible	meeting requirements to receive insurance or other types of benefits

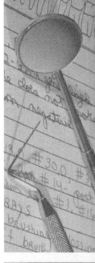

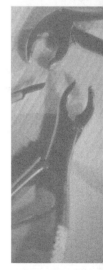

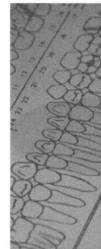

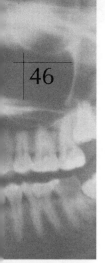
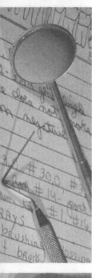
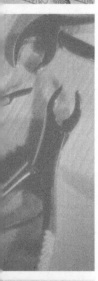
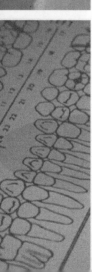

e

eliminate	to do away with
elongation	radiographic exposure error where the teeth appear to be greater in length than they actually are due to improper beam placement; too little vertical angulation
embedded	fixed securely in bone or tissue
embezzlement	stealing money from one's employer for one's own benefit
embrasure	V-shaped area located between the contact points of two teeth at the gingival crest
emphysema	condition of the lungs characterized by labored breathing and an increased susceptibility to infection
emulsion	radiation-sensitive coating on a radiographic film
enamel	substance that covers the anatomical crown of a tooth to protect the dentin; hardest substance in the human body
enamel rod	column that extends through the enamel and is perpendicular to the surface of the tooth
encephalitis	an infection characterized by swelling of the brain
endocarditis	an infection leading to inflammation of the heart valve and the membrane that lines the heart
endodontic explorer	often a double-ended instrument that is long and straight, used to locate canal openings
endodontic plugger	long, flat-ended instrument used to condense gutta-percha points in the root canal in a vertical direction
endodontics	branch of dentistry that is concerned with the morphology, physiology and pathology of the human dental pulp and periradicular tissues; its study and practice encompass the basic and clinical sciences including biology of the normal pulp, the etiology, diagnosis, prevention and treatment of diseases and injuries of the pulp and associated periradicular conditions
endodontic spreader	instrument used to spread gutta-percha in a lateral direction while filling the root canals
endodontist	dentist that specializes in performing endodontic treatments (root canals)
endospore	structures formed by some species of bacteria which are resistant to harsh environmental conditions

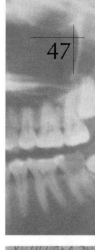

endogenous	originating from within the tooth
engineering controls	the Occupational Health and Safety Administration (OSHA) identifies these as any device that will isolate or remove Bloodborne pathogen hazards from the workplace; examples would include disposable scalpels and motion-sensitive water faucets
envelope flap	procedure performed in conjunction with osseous surgery; a tissue flap created by making a horizontal incision without a vertical incision
EOB	see explanation of benefit
EPA	acronym for the Environmental Protection Agency; see Appendix A
epiglottis	cartilage that is covered by mucous membrane that forms the superior part of the larynx and guards the glottis during swallowing
epilepsy	a disorder of cerebral function characterized by sudden recurring attacks of motor, sensory, or psychic malfunction with or without loss of consciousness and convulsions
epinephrine	vasoconstrictor that is added to some local anesthetics to enhance the therapeutic effect
epistaxis	bleeding from the nose
epithelial attachment	portion of the gingival sulcus that adheres to the surface of the teeth at or near the cementoenamel junction; junctional epithelium
epulis	tumor (tumescence) of the gingiva
ergonomics	study of body positioning and motion factors that affect a worker's heath, productivity, and mental well being
erosion	wearing away of teeth or restorations by chemical means
erupt	movement of teeth through the gingival tissues into the oral cavity
erythema	red or inflamed skin caused by capillary congestion
erythromycin	broad-spectrum antibiotic used for the treatment of mild infections
erythroplakia	any red patch of tissue in the oral cavity that cannot be associated with inflammation
esthetic	related to appearance and beauty; treatment for cosmetic purposes

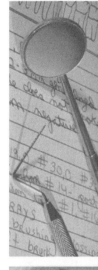

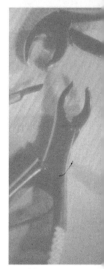

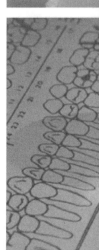

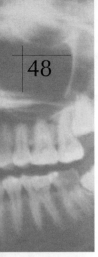

e

etchant (conditioner)	acid solution, usually phosphoric acid, used to decalcify or make microscopic undercuts between the enamel rods to allow for mechanical retention for the bonding of restorative materials
etiology	the cause assigned; the study of the cause or origin of disease
ethylene oxide	gas used at room temperature to sterilize instruments, equipment, and other materials that would otherwise be damaged by exposure to heat or liquid chemicals
ethics	a system of moral principles or practices; used to define what is normally right or wrong
eugenol	liquid from clove oil that has a palliative effect on the pulp of a tooth
evacuation system	vacuum system that uses suction to remove debris and fluids from the oral cavity through the use of high volume, high velocity and low pressure suction
evaporate	to fade away; to change from a solid or liquid state to a gaseous (vapor) state
excavation	to remove by scooping out
excessive	extreme; to exceed the norm
excision	act of cutting away or taking out
exclusion	dental services not provided under a dental plan
exempt	free from obligation; not required to fulfill any type of obligation
exfoliate	to shed teeth; typically referring to primary teeth
exogenous	originating outside of the tooth
exostosis	an enlargement or bony outgrowth (thin structure of bone extended from the facial surface) that appears on the facial surface of the mandible and the maxillary palate
exothermic reaction	chemical reaction that creates heat, resulting in setting of gypsum and other products
expanded functions	procedures dental assistants are legally allowed to perform in a particular state that often require an increased level of skill and responsibility, education and/or training or credentials
expectorate	to spit

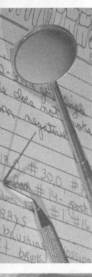

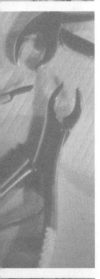

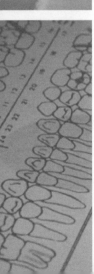

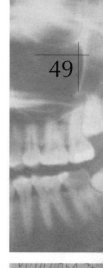

e

expiration date	date marked on various types of packages indicating the last date that product should be used; i.e. for radiographs it is the date that the manufacturer can no longer guarantee that the film might have been affected by normally existing background radiation
explanation of benefit (EOB)	statement from an insurance company that explains what procedures have been paid, the amount, and the procedures that have been denied coverage
explorer	double- or single-ended instrument with a slender, pointed working end used during an examination for the evaluation of pits and fissures, decay, root surfaces, and margins of existing amalgam, composite and cast restorations
exposed film	film that has been exposed to radiation or light

exposure
1) measure of gamma radiation to which a person is exposed
2) opening into the pulp of a tooth through mechanical means or decay process
3) when dental healthcare personnel (DHCP) come in contact with a patient's blood or other potentially infectious materials (OPIM)

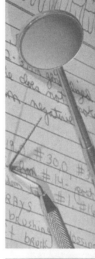

exposure control plan	written plan required of each office by the Occupational Safety and Health Administration's (OSHA's) Hazard Communication Standard; describes how employers will assure health care workers are protected from pathogens and hazardous materials
exposure management	the Occupational Safety and Health Administration (OSHA) identifies these as steps followed in the event of an accidental exposure to bloodborne pathogens; including first aid treatment, advanced medical treatment, immediate incident reporting, and referral for counseling
exposure time	amount of time a radiograph or person is exposed to radiation
external oblique line	slanted, bony growth line on the facial side of the mandible
external oblique ridge	anatomical structure that extends from the mental foramen, runs the length of the mandible and past the last tooth up to the ramus
external pterygoid muscle	one of the muscles of mastication that opens the jaw and thrusts the mandible forward
extirpation	to root out; cleaning out of nerve and pulp tissues found in root canal during therapy

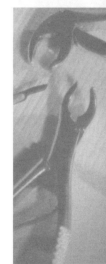

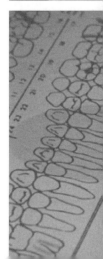

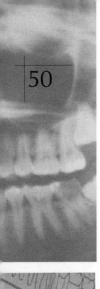

e

extract	to remove a tooth by use of elevators and/or forceps
extraction	intentional removal of a tooth
extraction elevators	see elevators
extraoral	outside of the mouth; frequently used in reference to orthodontic appliances that extend outside of the mouth; dental radiographs such as panoramic and cephalometric exposures
extraoral cassette	see cassette
extraoral exam	examination of the external head and neck structures for any abnormalities in relation to asymmetry, lesions, swellings, and discoloration through visual observance and palpation of external tissues
extraoral radiography	radiographs exposed outside of the oral cavity, such a panoramic and cephalometric exposures
extrinsic	external; on the outer surface of the teeth
extrude	1) to push or thrust out 2) retrognathic; Class II malocclusion, where the lower jaw is more distally placed 3) excessive eruption on a tooth beyond the line of occlusion
exudate	substance in liquid form which escaped from blood vessels usually as a result of inflammation; pus (purulent) or tissue (serous) fluid

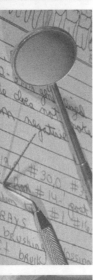

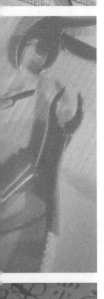

f

fabricate	to make
facebow	device used to record the relationship between the maxilla and temporomandibular joints
face mask	barrier used to cover the mouth and nose of dental healthcare personnel (DHCP) to filter splatter and aerosol from saliva and/or blood
facial surface	outer surface of; surface closest to the lips in the anterior and the cheeks in the posterior
facilitate	make easy; assist
Fair Credit Reporting Act	federal act that requires that the patient be informed of the reason for denial of credit and the name of the bureau from which the credit report was obtained
Fair Debt Collection Practices Act	enacted to protect a debtor from unfair collection practices by a dentist or collection agency

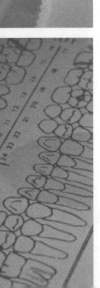

Fair Labor Standard Act	federal act prohibiting discrimination against individuals in the basis of gender, age, handicap, race, religion and national origin
FDA	acronym for the Food and Drug Administration; see Appendix A
felt wheel	device used to polish removable appliances and prosthetics
femoral artery	artery located in the thigh
fentanyl	narcotic analgesic used for the treatment of acute or chronic pain; generic name for Sublimaze®

festoon
1) carving in the base of a denture that simulates the contours of the natural tissues
2) lines in a crown designed to follow a line parallel to the gingival crest
3) curving of an orthodontic band or referring to the curving of the cervical line of a temporary crown

fiber bundles	group of fibers (such as those that support the tooth in the socket)
fibroblasts	immature fiber producing cells that are capable of developing connective tissue; found in tooth pulp
fibroma	benign tumor made primarily of fibrous connective tissue
fibrous	having a consistency similar to fibers; containing fibers
file, bone	instrument used to smooth the alveolus after extraction(s)
file, endodontic	hand or rotary instrument with spiraled blades used to clean and shape root canals in an endodontic procedure

Types
K-type–	used in the initial debridement of the canal and to shape and contour the canals
Headstrom–	used for final enlargement of the canal
Broaches–	barbed instrument used to remove the pulp tissue
Peeso–	used when a tooth needs a post-preparation
Lentulo spiral–	twisted instrument used in a low-speed handpiece or by hand, to place sealers or cements into the canals

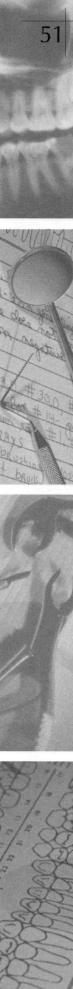

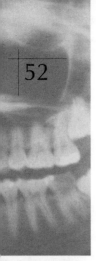

f

filiform	finger-like
filiform papillae	see papillae
film badge	see dosimeter
film packet	water resistant, opaque, lightproof plastic covering that contains lead foil, black paper, and radiographic film
film size	intraoral radiographic film varies in sizes for different exposures

0– pedodontic
1– anterior and vertical bitewings
2– bitewing and adult posterior periapical
3– can be used for adult bitewing
4– occlusal

film speed	how quickly a film will accept radiation; speed of radiographic film that is determined by the amount of radiation needed to produce a radiograph; depends on the size of the crystal on the radiographic film
filtration	removal of low-energy; long-wavelength x-rays that may be absorbed into the body but are not necessary for producing a radiograph
financial agreement	arrangements agreed upon between the patient and dentist for payment of services before treatment is initiated
financial ledger	record of debits and credits pertaining to all financial transactions for a patient
fissure	incomplete closure of a natural depression or developmental groove in the enamel of a tooth; usually an incomplete closing of the two parts resulting in an area of greater decay potential
fistula	tract leading from an abscess to the an external surface through which an abscess drains
fixer	radiographic solution that removes the unexposed and undeveloped crystals from the film emulsion and stops the developing process
fixing	hardening of the emulsion and preservation of the radiographic image on film
flash	excess material; i.e., restorative material from around a matrix
flora	bacteria that live in various parts of the body

Types
resident– normally found in that part of the body, such as in the oral cavity (normal oral flora)

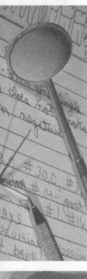

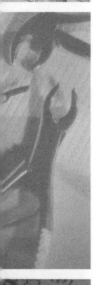

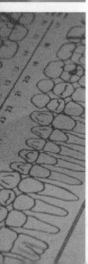

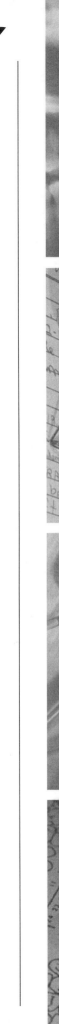

flora *(continued)*	**transient–**	when bacteria attach to a part of the body for a short period of time; lasting or staying only a short time
floss		see dental floss
flow		viscosity of any material
fluoride		natural mineral nutrient that can be applied topically to teeth to resist tooth decay
	1.23% acidulated phosphate–	applied for one to four minutes at six to twelve month intervals, most widely used fluoride solution, does not stain teeth
	2% sodium–	applied for three minutes at one-week intervals for four weeks, also used as a desensitizing agent for dentin
	8% stannous–	aqueous solution that must be prepared immediately before application. Causes discoloration of teeth because of the tin content.
fluoride rinse		over the counter solution that contains a concentration of .05% sodium fluoride that is used on a daily basis; prescription solutions contain a .63% stannous fluoride and 2% sodium fluoride
fluoride supplement		fluoride prescribed to patients that may not live in an area that receives fluoridated water, taken internally
fluoride trays		trays used to hold fluoride solutions for in-office administration of topical fluoride
fluorosis		condition caused by excessive ingestion of fluoride during the tooth development stage; teeth appear mottled and discolored
flush		to rinse with a water syringe or syringe filled with water; to run water through water lines in order to remove bioburden
FMX		acronym for full mouth x-rays; see full mouth series of radiographs
fog (fogging)		a grayish appearance to dental x-ray film
	Types **chemical–**	caused by an imbalance or breakdown of processing solutions
	radiation–	due to exposure to radiation from sources other than primary beam
foliate papillae		see papillae

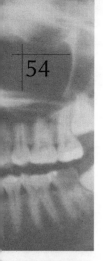

f

follicular (dentigerous) cyst	cyst that encloses the crown of an unerupted tooth and attaches near the cementoenamel junction
foramen	1) natural opening in the bone 2) opening at or near the apex of the tooth
forceps	1) hinged instrument used for the removal of teeth 2) instrument used to hold tissues, suture needles or small items
Fordyce's granuloma	sebaceous (oil) glands on the surface of epithelium; a common deviation from normal; multiple yellow round structures found in oral mucosa appearing just below the surface most often on the buccal mucosa
forensic dentistry	area of dentistry that deals with legal proceedings; including identifying deceased individuals through the use of dental radiographs, existing restorations and pathology
foreshortening	radiographic exposure error causing the teeth to appear shorter in length than they actually are due to improper beam placement; too much vertical angulation
formaldehyde	chemical used as a disinfectant or tissue preservative
formocreosol	chemical placed on the remaining exposed portion of the pulp during a pulpotomy procedure to prevent deterioration of the pulp
fossa	depression such as that found on the lingual surfaces of anterior and occlusal surfaces of posterior teeth, as well as on the surface of the bone
four-handed dentistry	chairside dentistry that makes efficient use of a dentist and a chairside assistant, where all four hands are kept busy working in and assisting with procedures in the oral cavity
framework	skeleton portion of a removable partial denture made of a metal alloy
Frankel appliance	see functional appliance
Frankfort plane	imaginary line from the bottom of the eye socket to the top of the ear that is parallel to the floor
free gingival graft	procedure performed when there is a minimal amount of gingival tissue around teeth; a small strip of tissue is removed from the roof of the mouth and sutured to the existing gingival tissue in the area being treated

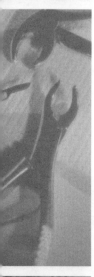

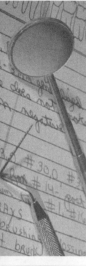

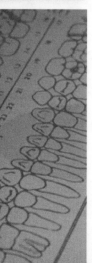

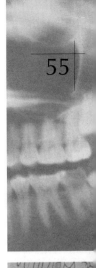

freeze dried bone	see bone substitute
frenectomy	surgical procedure performed to detach the frenum
frenum	tissue attachments that extend from the alveolar mucosa to the vestibule and are located on the maxillary and mandibular arches at the midline and on either side of each arch in the canine/premolar areas; the lingual frenum attaches the tongue to the floor of the mouth
friction	rubbing of one object against another; can cause build up of heat
fulcrum	position of stabilization for the fingers when using a handpiece or hand instrument
full mouth series of radiographs	a series of radiographs consisting of periapical and bitewing radiographs that provides a survey of the entire mouth
functional appliance	removable orthodontic appliance used to change the direction of growth or inhibit the growth rate of one arch while the teeth and cranial-facial skeleton are still developing
fungi	group of organisms, one of which is the cause of candidiasis
fungiform papillae	see papillae
furcation	point where the roots of a multi-rooted tooth separate
fusiform bacillus	microorganism that is thought to be a factor in causing necrotizing ulcerative gingivitis

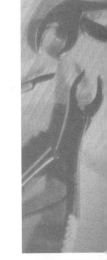

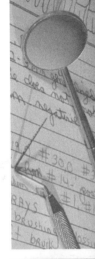

gag reflex	involuntary action caused by touching something to the posterior palate or throat area
galvanic reaction	having an electrical effect; shock-type symptoms that occur when restorations of different materials on opposite arches come in contact with each other; for this reaction to occur the pH level in the mouth has to be acidic
gamma radiation	see radiation
gasket	rubber or rubber-like material placed around the door of sterilization equipment to create an impenetrable seal so that the sterilization process will not be compromised
gastrointestinal	relates to the stomach and intestines
gauze	thin, sterile cotton fabric with a loose weave

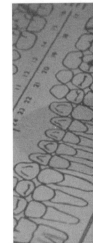

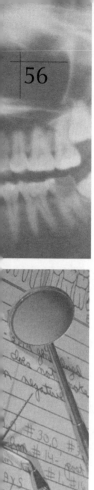
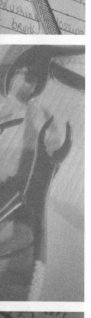

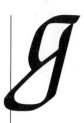

GC	acronym for the national DANB General Chairside component exam
Gelfoam®	surgical sponge placed in a socket immediately after a tooth has been removed
general practitioner	dentist who practices all types of dentistry
general supervision	see supervision
genetic	reproductive cells; cells containing DNA
genetic changes	changes in future generations due to chromosome damage
genial tubercles	small, rounded projections and raised areas on the inner surface of the mandible that serve as attachments for the genioglossus and geniohyoid muscles; are critical landmarks for the subperiosteal implant
genioglossus muscle	muscle that depresses and protrudes the tongue
geniohyoid muscle	muscle that elevates and protracts hyoid bone; depresses the mandible
geographic tongue	temporary loss of papillae from the surface of the tongue; areas of loss migrate around the dorsal surface of the tongue from tip to root
germicidal	agent with ability to kill a variety of microorganisms
ghost image	a fault in a dental radiograph that is seen when a radiopaque image in superposed onto the film from a high-density object such as glasses or earrings
gingiva	fibrous tissue that surrounds the necks of the teeth and covers the alveolar processes; healthy gingiva is pink, firm and stippled
gingival grafting	procedure where gingival tissue is taken from one area in the mouth and placed on another
gingival crest	top of the free gingiva
gingival hyperplasia	overgrowth of gingival tissue often caused by plaque, orthodontic braces and a variety of drugs, especially Dilantin®
gingival margin trimmer	instrument with a curved, angled blade used to trim the gingival margin of a cavity preparation
gingival recession	loss of gingival tissue causing exposure of the cementum
gingivectomy	surgical removal of unattached and/or diseased gingival tissue
gingivitis	inflammation of the gingiva associated with poor oral hygiene, smoking and emotional stress

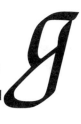

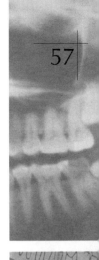

gingivoplasty	reshaping of the gingival tissue to remove deformities
gingivostomatitis	inflammation of the gingival and oral mucosa; can be caused by herpes virus; membraneous gingivostomatitis forms on the givgiva and oral mucosa leaving a raw and bleeding surface
glass ionomer cement	permanent fluoride releasing cement used for cementation of permanent restorations and endodontic posts; as a liner in Class I, II, III, and V restorations; for restoring cervical erosions, root caries and Class III and V cavities
glass slab	sheet of glass used to mix dental materials
glenoid fossa	depression in the temporal bone within which the condyles of the mandible articulate
glottis	anatomical area located in the back of the throat; part of larynx that contains the vocal cords
gloves	PPE used as a barrier to microorganisms

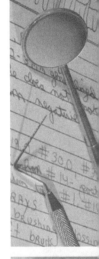

Types
exam gloves–gloves worn as a barrier from microorganisms

procedure/ exam–	single use, non-sterile, disposable latex or non-latex gloves worn during all patient care activities where there is a potential for direct contact with saliva, blood, or other oral fluids, mucous membranes, and nonintact skin, and when handling items or surfaces contaminated with body fluids or potentially infectious materials
sterile or surgical–	individually packaged as a set with a right-hand glove and a left -hand glove; intended for single use during specific surgical procedures
utility–	gloves that are thicker and used during disinfection and cleanup procedures
nitrile–	much like utility gloves; however, an added benefit is that they can be sterilized in the autoclave after use
latex–	rubber-based gloves that are ambidextrous, used interchangeably for the right or left hand; made of natural rubber; see procedure/exam

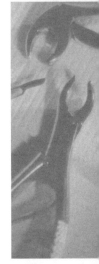

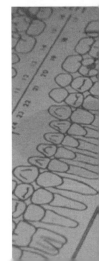

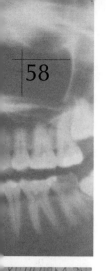

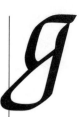

gloves *(continued)*   **vinyl–**   synthetic material more rigid than latex, therefore tearing more easily and lacking the tactile sensitivity; used when latex-sensitivity is a concern

glucose   most important carbohydrate in body metabolism; also known as dextrose

glutaraldehyde   liquid used for high level disinfection and sterilization of dental instruments

gold   precious metal used for permanent restorations; i.e., crowns, inlays, onlays

gonad   an ovary or testis; the site or origin of eggs and spermatozoa; relates to tissues involved in reproduction

graft   removing tissue or bone from one site and relocating it to another

<u>Types</u>
autogenous– graft of bone or other tissue taken from one portion of an individual's body and implanted into another part

free–   tissue detached from its orginal site and moved to another area

pedicle–   gingival tissue is raised from the area immediately lateral to an area of recession and is rotated over the area of recession while leaving the tissue attached at the base

grand mal seizure   a medical emergency characterized by unconsciousness, jerking of the body, twitching, and stiffening

granulation tissue   soft, pink fleshy projections that form during the healing process in a wound

granuloma   tumor that is filled with granulation tissue

grinding wheel   wheel on a model trimmer used to shape plaster or stone models/casts

gross income   total of accounts receivable before accounts payable totals are subtracted

gutta percha   plastic-type material that is made from exudates from sap trees mixed with lime, quartz and feldspar; used as a temporary stopping material, thermal conductor for pulp testing, and to obdurate (fill) canals in an endodontic treatment

gypsum   material used to fabricate models for various uses

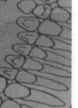

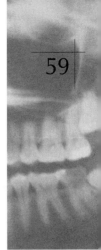

HA	acronym for horizontal angle
halitosis	bad breath
hamular process	projection of bone that is located posterior and medial to the maxillary tuberosity
hand hygiene	procedures related to handwashing, alcohol-based handscrub and surgical hand hygiene/antisepsis
handpiece	rotary instrument that is powered by compressed air or electricity to rotate burs, discs, and stones

Types

contra–angle–	attachment used on a low speed handpiece to hold burs, discs, stones, polishing cups and brushes that have latch type shanks
high-speed–	handpiece used for rapid cutting of tooth structure; rotates between 100,000 and 500,000 rpm
low-speed–	handpiece used to polish teeth and restorations, remove decay; rotates between 6,000 and 25,000 rpm
right-angle–	attachment for use with prophylaxis cups or brushes
straight–	slow-speed handpiece used without any attachments for long-shank mandrels and friction grip laboratory burs

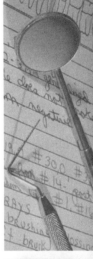

hand washing	washing hands with plain (i.e., nonantimicrobial) soap and water
hardware	equipment used by a computer system; houses software
hard x-rays	description of an x-ray as a function of wavelength; the shorter the wavelength, the harder the x-ray
HAV	hepatitis A virus; see hepatitis
Hawley retainer	see retainer
Hazard Communication Standard	Occupational Safety and Health Administration (OSHA) guideline that requires dental offices to develop and implement a program to instruct all employees who might be exposed to hazardous materials in the safe handling and disposal of those materials (For a copy of the Standard, go to www.osha.gov.)

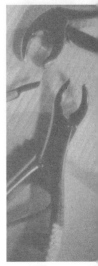

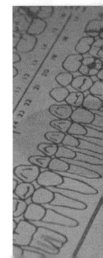

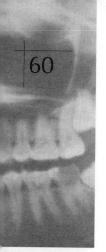

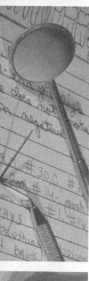

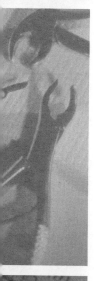

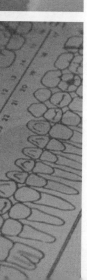

h

hazardous material	material that could cause damage or harm peoples' health; can be caustic to tissue, respiratory systems, the environment; may be flammable
HBV	hepatitis B virus; see hepatitis
HCAI	acronym for healthcare associated infections
HCV	hepatitis C virus; see hepatitis
HDV	hepatitis D virus; see hepatitis
headgear	an orthodontic appliance that encircles the head or neck and has an intraoral attachment; used to aid in tooth movement

Types

cervical–	designed for the treatment of mandibular retrognathism and/or maxillary prognathism, particularly with respect to patients diagnosed with Class II, deep bite tendencies
reverse pull–	designed for treatment of maxillary insufficiencies, mandibular prognathism, palatal schisis and generally for hinder-front tractions
Class III–	allows forward pull to bring maxillary arch forward
Class II–	allows forward pull on the mandibular arch; excellent for bringing teeth (individual or sections) forward
high pull face crib–	designed for the treatment of mandibular retrognathism and/or maxillary prognathism, particularly with respect to patients diagnosed with Class II, open bite tendencies

health history	information provided by a patient describing past and present health conditions; describes medications being taken and family medical conditions
Health Maintenance Organization (HMO)	health care delivery system that utilizes group practices and provides alternatives to fee-for-service practice
heat labile	readily changed or broken down by heat
heat sensitive	affected or damaged by heat
heat resistant	not affected or damaged by heat

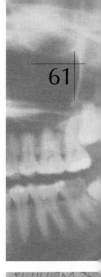

Heimlich maneuver application of thrusts to the abdomen forcing air from the diaphragm to expel a blockage in the airway

hematoma bruise; may result intraorally from a mandibular block injection that has ruptured a blood vessel; see ecchymosis

hemisection complete sectioning of a tooth into the furcation through the crown for the surgical removal of one root of a tooth

hemostasis to control or stop the flow of blood; this can be done by using instruments to clamp blood vessels by applying pressure, or by using chemicals

hemoglobin iron containing pigment of the red blood cells used to carry oxygen from the lungs to the tissues

hemorrhage excessive bleeding from blood vessels

hemostat 1) instrument used to carry, hold or manipulate small objects
2) a chemical used to stop the flow of blood

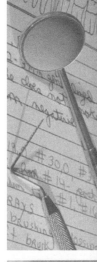

hepatitis disease resulting in an inflammation of the liver; is transmitted and contracted by human serum or through contaminated food or water

Types

hepatitis A (HAV)– spread by the fecal/oral route, typically through contaminated food and water

hepatitis B (HBV)– bloodborne disease that can be transmitted by body fluids and destroys liver cells, may lead to cirrhosis of the liver and death

hepatitis C (HCV)– typically transmitted through blood transfusions or percutaneous exposure to blood

hepatitis D (HDV)– virus that cannot replicate itself without the presence of HBV

hepatitis E (HEV)– typically transmitted through the fecal/oral route from contaminated food and water

hepatitis G (HGV)– is transmitted through bloodborne routes and frequently occurs as a co-infection with HCV

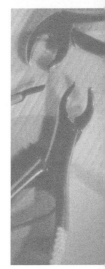

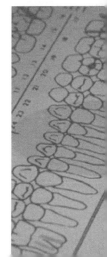

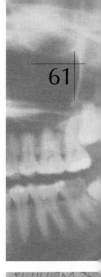

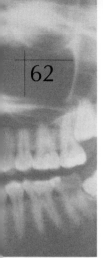

h

Herbst appliance	fixed or removable appliance designed to enhance the growth of the mandible in a forward direction while applying pressure to the maxillae in a backward direction
hereditary	genetic traits transmitted from parent to child, ancestor to ancestor
herpes simplex	viral infection that most often occurs initally in patients between the ages of 2 and 5 that may present as acute herpetic gingivostomatitis, keratoconjunctivitis, vulvovaginitis, or encephalitis; recurrent manifestations include fever blisters or cold sores
herpetic gingivostomatitis	inflammation of the gingiva and mucosa caused by herpes virus occurring typically in pediatric patients that lasts for approximately 14 days; characteristics are red and swollen gingiva, red mucosa with painful vesicles and ulcers
herringbone pattern	radiographic image that has a fish-bone or tire track appearance created by the lead foil in an x-ray packet when the radiographic film is placed in the mouth backward and exposed
HEV	hepatitis E virus; see hepatitis
HGV	hepatitis G virus; see hepatitis
high speed handpiece	see handpiece
high volume evacuation	system used to remove fluids and debris in order to maintain a clear, dry operating field
HIPAA	acronym for Health Insurance Portability and Accountability Act
histamine	substance stored in and released from mast cells of the immune system during an allergic response
histology	the study of tissues
HIV	see human immudeficiency virus
HMO	see Health Maintenance Organization
holding solution	disinfectant, or even soapy water used to soak instruments until the sterilization process can be completed; prevents debris from drying on the instruments
homogenous bone	graft of bone taken from a donor and transplanted into the patient
horizontal	parallel to, in the plane of, or operating in a plane parallel to the horizon or to a base line
horizontal angulation	direction of the central beam of radiation through interproximal spaces

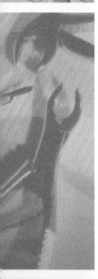

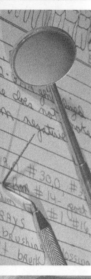

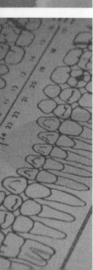

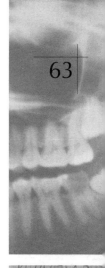

housekeeping surfaces	surfaces (i.e., floors, walls and sinks) with limited risk of disease transmission that can be decontaminated with less rigorous methods than those used on dental patient-care items and clinical contact surfaces
Howe pliers	instrument used to make archwire and ligature adjustments
human immunodeficiency virus (HIV)	bloodborne or sexually transmitted viral infection that substantially compromises the immune system; is the cause of Acquired Immunodeficiency Syndrome (AIDS)
humidor	container used to store materials at a constant level of humidity
Hutchinson's incisors	defect in tooth development resulting in shorter than normal incisors with a single permanent notch in each incisal edge; may be caused by congenital syphilis
HVE	see high volume evacuation
hydrocolloid	agar-based impression material that can be reversible and irreversible
hydrocortisone	steroid used to treat inflammation, endocrine (hormonal) disorders, many immune and allergic disorders, arthritis, lupus, severe psoriasis and asthma, ulcerative colitis, Crohn's disease
hydrogen peroxide	oxidizing liquid used as a mild antiseptic; in higher concentrations can be used as a tooth bleaching solution
hydroxyapatite	inorganic component of bone, teeth and calculus that is used as a replacement for bone; it forms a lattice-work for bone formation
hyperemia	excessive amounts of blood in the tissues
hyperglycemia	increase in the concentration of sugar in the blood above normal levels
hyperkinetic	neurological disorder characterized by increased muscular movement; common movement disorders may include tremors, tics and Tourette's syndrome
hyperplasia	abnormal multiplication of normal cells resulting in a thickening or enlargement of the tissue
hyperplastic	relating to hyperplasia; i.e., excessive moveable tissue on the maxilla or mandible resulting from an increase in the number of normal cells
hypertension	higher than normal blood pressure; usually blood pressure that is 140/90 or higher; hypertensive patients are often asymptomatic

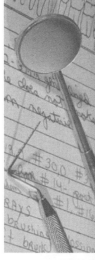

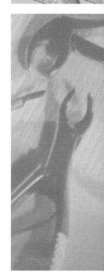

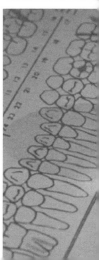

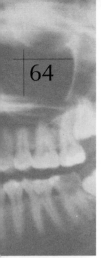

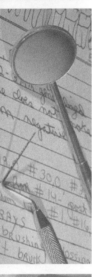

h

hyperthyroidism	condition caused from excessive activity of the thyroid gland characterized by weight loss, fatigue, insomnia, fast or irregular heartbeat, shortness of breath, chest pain and muscle weakness
hypertrophy	to grow abnormally large
hyperventilation	rapid, deep breathing with a decrease in carbon dioxide; may cause confusion, dizziness, tingling of fingers, numbness, decrease in blood pressure and possibility of syncope
hypocalcification	undercalcified enamel
hypoglossal nerve	motor nerve that supplies extrinsic and intrinsic muscles of the tongue
hypoglycemia	abnormally low level of sugar in the blood
hypoplasia	incomplete development of tooth enamel
hyposensitive	below normal ability to respond to stimuli
hypotension	arterial blood pressure below normal; patients treated for hypotension may experience sudden drop in blood pressure when standing up quickly (postural hypotension), resulting in symptoms of faintness, dizziness, confusion, blurry vision and passing out
hypoxemia	insufficient oxygenation of the blood
hypoxia	insufficient amount of oxygen

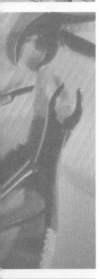

i

ICE	acronym for the national DANB Infection Control component exam
ICO	see infection control officer
immediate dentures	dentures inserted directly after the teeth are extracted
immerse	to completely cover with liquid
immune	unable to contract a disease; able to resist/not susceptible to infection
immunize	to render immune
immunocompromised	condition in which the functioning of the immune system is reduced or incapable of protecting the body
impacted	tooth that is wedged in place or at an angle that does not allow it to erupt

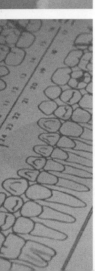

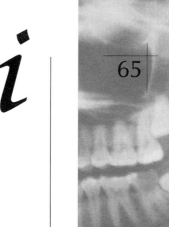

impingement	excessive pressure placed on tissues by removable prosthesis, provisional or permanent restoration or dental dam clamp
implant	single unit fixed prosthesis that is surgically placed in the maxilla or mandible to replace a missing tooth/teeth or used to support a bar for the attachment of a denture
implied consent	consent to treatment given by a patient's actions, rather than in writing
impregnated	saturated
impregnated retraction cord	see retraction cord
impression	negative reproduction of the maxillary and/or mandibular arches used for study casts, crown and bridge, etc.
inadvertent	accidental; unintentional
incipient	beginning decay that has not broken completely through the enamel into the dentin
incisal	cutting edge of the incisors and canines
incise	cut into
incisive foramen	opening located at the midline of the palate behind the central incisors
incisive papilla	elevation of tissue covering the foramen of the incisive canal located lingual to the maxillary central incisors
incisor	cutting tooth; there are two in each quadrant
incubator	apparatus used to provide a suitable atmospheric condition for culturing bacteria
indexing unit	letter by which a name or word is filed or placed into alphabetical order
indicator tape	tape applied to the outside of instrument packaging which will change color rapidly when a specific parameter (temperature) is reached and verify that the package has been exposed to the sterilization process
indirect exposure	transmission of microorganisms from one person to another due to improper sterilization or handling techniques, touching contaminated surfaces and then touching the face, eyes, or mouth
indirect pulp cap	see pulp capping
indirect supervision	see supervision
infection	invasion of the body by disease producing microorganisms

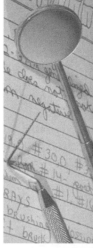

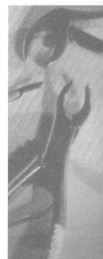

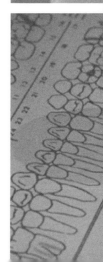

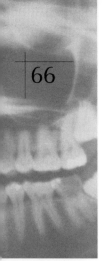

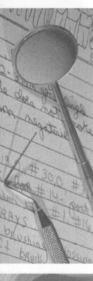

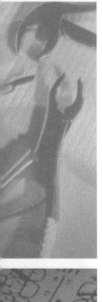

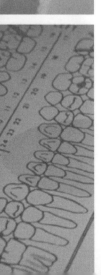

66

i

infection control	protocol employed to minimize the transmission of infectious microorganisms
infection control officer (ICO)	dental healthcare personnel (DHCP) assigned the responsibility of managing office safety and compliance with the Occupational Safety and Health Administration (OSHA) standards; see safety officer
inferior alveolar nerve	largest branch of the mandibular nerve; provides nerve supply to the mandibular teeth and mandibular anterior gingival tissue
infiltration injection	see injection
inflammation	reaction of tissue due to injury, irritation, or infection characterized by redness, pain and swelling
influenza	viral infection commonly known as the flu
ingestion	to take into the system by swallowing
inhalation	the act of breathing into the lungs
inhibit	to restrain
injectable	ability to be introduced into the body by needle
injection	introduction of a liquid substance into the body (via bloodstream or tissue) by needle

Types
block– also referred to as a field or mandibular block; this technique has the anesthetic solution being deposited at or near a major terminal nerve

infiltration– process where by anesthetic is deposited onto tissue and allowed to be absorbed by the nerve endings

intraligamentary– this technique uses pressure to inject the anesthetic solution into the periodontal membrane of specific teeth

inlay	gold, porcelain or resin restoration that is placed between the cusps of a tooth
inoculate	to inject a person with a microorganism or other antigenic material to immunize against disease
insoluble	will not dissolve

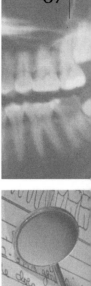

instrument grasp	different ways to place the fingers and palm to hold instruments

<u>Types</u>

pen grasp–	holding an instrument at the junction of the shank and handle like that of a pen or pencil
modified pen grasp –	holding an instrument like the pen grasp except the pad of the middle finger is placed on top of the instrument with the index finger
palm grasp–	holding the instrument in the palm of the hand, using the palm and fingers to grasp the handle of the instrument
palm-thumb grasp–	holding the instrument in the palm of the hand with the four fingers wrapped around the handle with the thumb extended upward
reverse palm-thumb grasp–	used to hold evacuator tip in the palm of the hand with the thumb directed toward the assistant instead of the patient; occasionally used to hold instruments

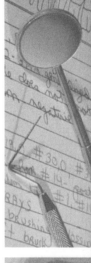

instrument transfer	the removal of a used instrument at the same time as a new instrument is placed into the operator's hand
insufficient funds	not enough money in a checking or savings account to cover an amount withdrawn; see nonsufficient funds (NSF)
insulin	substance normally produced by the body that is essential for metabolism of glucose to maintain a proper blood sugar (glucose) level
insurance carrier	insurance company
insurance claim form	form that includes demographic information for both the dentist and patient, date of treatment, procedure(s) completed and fees charged for that patient; submitted to the insurance company for reimbursment

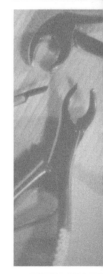

intact	unimpaired; unaltered; unbroken
intensifying screen	extraoral radiographic cassette component that increases the action of the x-rays through the use phosphor on the screen
interdental	between the teeth
interdental papilla	triangular shaped gingiva that fills in the space between the teeth in the area beneath the contact points

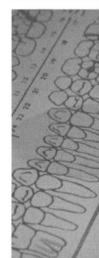

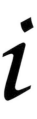

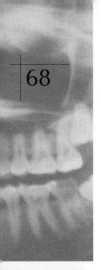

i

interface	point at which two things are joined, such as the joining of computer systems and programs or a restoration and the surface of the tooth
inter-maxillary	between the maxilla and mandible
intermediate restorative material	reinforced zinc oxide-eugenol (ZOE) composition used as a short term restoration or can be used for permanent cementation; i.e., IRM®
internal pterygoid muscle	muscle of mastication that raises the mandible to close the jaw
interproximal	between proximal surfaces of adjacent (touching) teeth
interproximal carver	instrument used to remove excess filling material from the gingival area of proximal restorations
interproximal space	space between adjacent teeth
intraligamentary injection	see injection
intra-maxillary	within the maxilla
intraoral radiography	exposing radiographs inside the oral cavity
intravascular	introduction of an agent into the blood vessels using a needle
intravenous	introduction of an agent into the body directly into a vein
intrinsic	internal; within the tooth; i.e., shade or staining
intubate	to insert a tube into a patient's airway
inventory	accurate physical count of supplies and equipment
Inverse Square Law	physics law that states that the intensity of radiation is inversely proportional to the square of the distance from the source of radiation; calculated by the following mathematical formula: original intensity over new intensity is equal to new distance squared over original distance squared
invert	to turn inside out or upside down
iodophor	liquid used as an intermediate-level disinfectant
ion	molecule that has one or more atoms possessing an electrical charge
irreversible hydrocolloid	impression material that cannot be returned to its original state
irrigant	solution used to flush debris from a root canal or wound

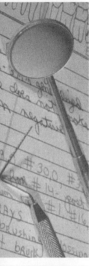

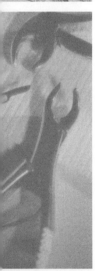

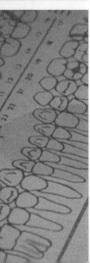

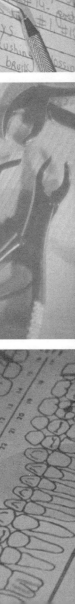

irrigation	act of flushing debris from a root canal or wound
irritant	caustic agent that causes irritation to tissue
ischemia	local and temporary anemia due to obstruction of the circulation to a part of the body
isolation	separate a person from another to prevent transmission of disease; separation of one area from another to prevent contamination
itemized charges	list of completed procedures and fees charged

jaundice	yellowish discoloration of tissue and body fluids caused by a pathological condition that interrupts normal processing of bile; can be associated with liver disease
JCAHO	acronym for Joint Commission on Accreditation of Healthcare Organizations
jurisprudence	the state laws covering the legal limitations of oral health care practice

Kaposi's sarcoma	1) neoplastic condition affecting blood vessels; believed to be of multicentric origin 2) unique cancer (malignancy) of blood vessels that is seen more often in AIDS patients
keratoconjunctivitis	inflammation of the cornea and the conjuctiva
kidney stones	stones formed from mineral salts in the body that can block the urinary tract; if left untreated, can cause loss of kidney function or rupture
kilovoltage	the difference in electric potential between the anode (negatively charged) and cathode (positively charged) in an x-ray tube
kilovoltage potential (kVp)	measurement that determines the penetrating power and quality of the radiation rays; determines contrast of a film
kVp	acronym for kilovoltage peak; see kilovoltage

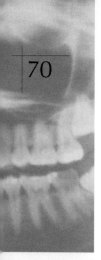

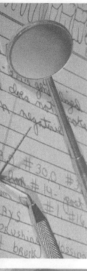

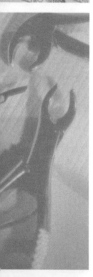

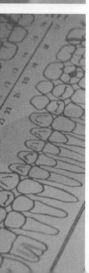

C

labial	surface of anterior teeth that is toward the lips
labial commissures	corners of the mouth where the upper and lower lips meet
laboratory requisition	form that indicates the name of the dentist, patient, date needed, what needs to be fabricated, materials to be used, shades, special instructions and signature of the dentist
lacerate	to cut or tear jaggedly
lactated Ringer's solution	specific intravenous solution used for rehydration
lamina dura	compact bone the lies adjacent to the periodontal membrane and lines the alveolar socket
laryngospasm	spasm of the larynx
larynx	anatomical structure used to produce the voice
latent image	invisible image on a radiographic film caused by the action of light or radiation before development
latent period	time between radiologic exposure and the onset of somatic changes
lateral	position either to the right or to the left of something; to the side
lateral incisor	tooth distal to a central incisor; there are four lateral incisors present in the permanent and primary dentition
laterally displaced flap (pedicle)	incisional periodontal surgery performed to lift and slide gingival tissue to cover a root surface that has inadequate tissue coverage
lateral movement	movement of the head or mandible from side to side
latex	thick, milky juice from certain seed plants; material used in the manufacture of exam gloves and dental dam
lathe	laboratory equipment used to polish removable prostheses
lead apron	apron placed over the patient to reduce exposure of radiation; contains lead or lead equivalent materials
lead foil	material incorporated into a radiographic film packet to absorb most unused radiation and reduce the scattering of secondary radiation and film fogging
leakage radiation	radiation that emits in all directions from a malfunctioning tubehead

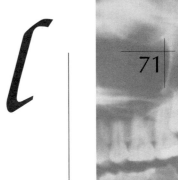

ledger card	accounting record for keeping track of debits, credits, and financial adjustments for a patient or family
lesion	an injury or wound; pathologic change of tissue resulting in loss of normal appearance or function
lethargic	sluggish; inactive
leukemia	types of cancer of the blood and hemopoietic tissue from an unknown origin that is characterized by rapid growth of leukocytes in the blood-forming organs; may result in death
leukocyte	white blood cell
leukoplakia	white spots or patches found on the oral mucous membrane; cannot be wiped off; cannot be diagnosed specifically
libel	writing something that will harm a reputation
lichen planus	a disease of unknown etiology which appears as a lacy pattern affecting the skin and oral mucous membrane, either alone or concomitantly (jointly); reticular form characterized by white lines that intersect in a lacy fashion and a circular pattern
lidocaine	local anesthetic; generic name for Xylocaine®

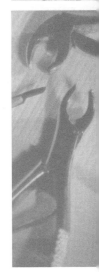

ligature	1)	floss or rubber material used to stabilize a dental dam or tied to a rubber dam clamp (retainer) to avoid aspiration should the clamp (retainer) pop off of the tooth and fall into the patient's throat
	2)	wire material used to secure an orthodontic archwire into the brackets
	3)	material used to bind teeth or to hold structures in place

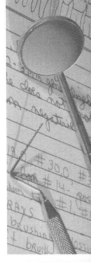

ligature cutter	instrument used to cut ligature wire
ligature director	instrument used to direct and place ligature wire ends into interproximal spaces or to guide elastic or wire ligature ties around a bracket
ligature locking plier	instrument used to apply and lock wire ligatures
ligature tie	wire or plastic device used to secure an archwire into an orthodontic bracket
ligature tucker	instrument used to guide a ligature and assist with bending wire edges
ligature tying pliers	instrument used to tie ligature wires
ligature wire	thin wire used to secure an archwire in a bracket
light-cure	see curing

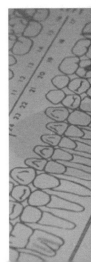

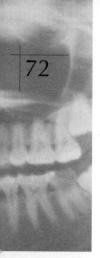

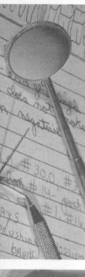

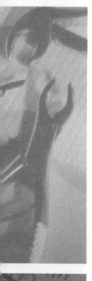

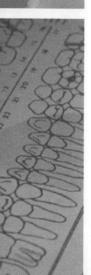

L

light-cured materials	materials that are hardened by means of a curing light; see curing
linea alba	raised white line on the buccal mucosa of the cheek that runs parallel to where the maxillary and mandibular teeth occlude
lingual	surface of a tooth, both maxillary and mandibular, adjacent to the tongue; see palatal
lingual braces	braces that are placed on the lingual surfaces of the teeth for esthetic purposes
lingual nerve	sensory branch of the mandibular nerve with sublingual and lingual branches
lipids	fats or fatlike substances (fatty acids, glycerol) that are insoluble in water
long axis	imaginary line that passes longitudinally (top to bottom) through the center of the tooth
loop forming pliers	instrument used to form and shape loops in orthodontic wires
lubricant	oil or grease agent used to reduce heat caused by friction in moving parts
luster	soft sheen or gloss
luting	1) bonding or cementing together 2) bonding agent with a consistency that is somewhat viscous and tends to be stringy like honey
luxate	to displace or dislocate a tooth from the socket; intentionally completed with extraction instruments
lymph node	mass of lymphoid tissue that form tissue which acts as a filter of bacteria
lymphadenopathy	any disease process that generally involves inflammation or draining of lymph node or nodes
lymphangioma	benign tumor of the lymph vessels
lymphoid tissue	lymph nodes, spleen, thymus and tonsils
lymphocytes	white blood cells formed in lymphoid tissue

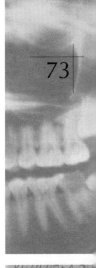

magnetic resonance imaging (MRI)	medical diagnostic technique that creates images of the body using the principles of nuclear magnetic resonance; generating thin-section images of any part of the body, including the heart, arteries, and veins from any angle and direction; without surgical invasion and in a relatively short period of time; used to diagnosis TMJ
magnification	enlarge the size or the reflection of an object
mail	to send something from one place or person to another through the U.S. Postal System or by independent carrier; i.e., Federal Express or United Parcel Service

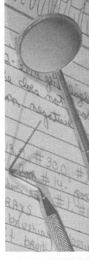

Definitions and types of items usually sent

first class–	letters, business reply mail, invoices
second class–	newspapers and magazines
third class–	books, catalogs
fourth class–	printed material and packages that weigh more than 16 ounces
special delivery–	available for all classes of mail; is delivered as soon as the post office receives it
certified mail–	available for first-class mail; sender is provided a receipt, and upon request, proof of delivery
insured mail–	for first class, priority, third and fourth class mail; may be insured up to a determined amount against damage, loss and theft
registered mail–	available for first-class mail; sender is provided a receipt and proof of delivery
special handling–	available for third and fourth class mail; receives fastest handling of third and fourth class mail
express mail–	mail is delivered within 24 hours
priority mail–	mail is delivered within 2 to 3 days

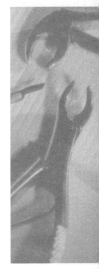

major treatment	dental treatment designation that includes crowns and bridges, implants, removable prosthetics, endodontics, periodontics, etc.
malar bone	see zygoma

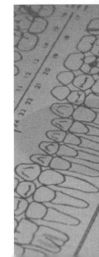

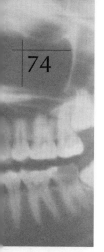
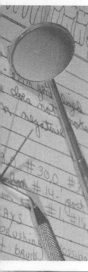
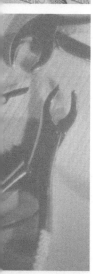
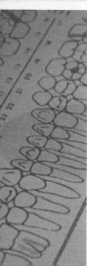

m

malignant	resistant to treatment; has the ability to kill the patient; usually used in reference to cancer
malleability	ability to change or be transformed; specifically ability of dental material to withstand compressive stresses without fracturing or rupturing
malocclusion	irregularities in the way the maxillary and mandibular teeth occlude

<u>Types</u>

anterior cross bite–	one or more of the maxillary incisors is positioned lingual to the opposing mandibular incisors
posterior cross bite–	one or more of the maxillary posterior teeth is positioned lingual to the mandibular teeth
edge-to-edge bite–	incisal surfaces of the maxillary anterior teeth meet the incisal surfaces of the mandibular anterior teeth
end-to-end bite–	maxillary posterior teeth meet the mandibular posterior teeth cusp-to-cusp
open bite–	insufficient overlap of the maxillary incisors creating an opening of the anterior teeth
overbite–	vertical projection of the upper t teeth over the lower
overjet–	horizontal projection of the upper teeth over the lower

malpositioned	out of alignment
malpractice	negligent treatment provided to a patient by a health care provider
mamelons	development divisions (tubercles) that appear as bulges on the incisal edges of newly erupted central and lateral incisors
mandible	lower arch
mandibular	refers to the lower arch
mandibular canal	houses the mandibular nerve and blood supply; extends from the mandibular foramen to the mental foramen
mandibular foramen	opening located on the mesial surface of each ramus posterior to the retromolar pad, that contains the inferior alveolar nerve

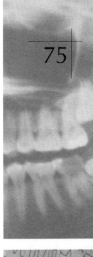

mandibular nerve	branch of the trigeminal nerve that registers sensation and causes movement in the mandibular arch
mandibular notch	structure located on the mandible, between the coronoid process and the condyle
mandrel	metal rod for the attachment of discs and stones; used in low-speed handpieces and polishing lathes
manipulate	to mix or handle; specifically, cements, dental stone, impression materials, etc.
manometer	mercury gravity gauge used to measure blood pressure
margin	point where a restoration meets tooth structure
marginal fracture	breakage of a restoration at the margin
marginal ridge	area of the enamel that forms the mesial or distal border or boundary of the occlusal surface of a tooth

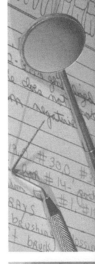

margination	1) the process of removing excess amalgam and overhangs; finishing all cavosurface margins to ensure continuous, uninterrupted, smooth relationships between restorative materials and tooth structure 2) molecular attraction of leukocytes (white blood cells) to the luminal (tube, cavity or passage in a tubular organ) surface of blood vessel walls in the early stages of inflammation
margin trimmer	see gingival margin trimmer
Maryland bridge	fixed bridge that replaces one tooth that is secured to the adjacent teeth with resin; requires minimal preparation of abutment teeth

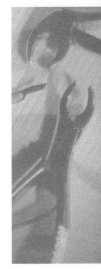

masseter muscle	muscle that closes the jaw
mastication	act of chewing that is aided by the teeth, tongue, maxilla, mandible, muscles, cheeks, and temporomandibular joints
materia alba	soft, white food debris and bacterial growth that collects in grooves and spaces on teeth, gingiva and appliances that provides a source for plaque growth

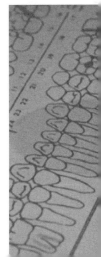

Material Safety Data Sheet (MSDS)	information provided by manufacturers of potentially hazardous products that must include product identification, chemical content, hazardous ingredients, physical data, fire and explosion information, reactivity data, health hazard data, emergency and first aid procedures, spill or leak procedures, labeling and storage

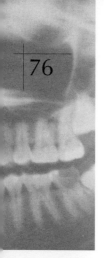

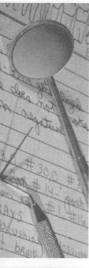

m

Mathieu needle holder	instrument used to tie ligature wires, place elastic ligatures and sutures
matrix	form placed around the parimeter of a tooth to replace a missing wall(s) so the restorative material will be confined upon placement and condensation
maxilla	upper arch
maxillary	refers to upper arch
maxillary nerve	branch of the trigeminal nerve registering sensation to the maxilla
maxillary sinus	opening or air space that extends from the canine or premolar region to the molar region; see sinus
maxillary tuberosity	rounded area of the maxilla behind the most posterior molar
maxillofacial	referring to the face and jaws, both maxilla and mandible
maximum permissible dose (MPD)	maximum amount of radiation a person can be exposed to over a stated period of time; limitation defined by the National and International Council on Radiation Protection and Measurement (NCRP)
measles	highly communicable virus that can cause inflammation of the mucous membranes; symptoms include: Koplik's spots, fever and skin lesions
mechanical bond	bond obtained when bonding solution flows into microscopic lattice-work of etched enamels and dentinal tubules and locks into place; unlike a chemical bond, no change in the structure of matter occurs
mechanical retention	retention obtained by cutting the walls of a preparation larger at the floor of the preparation than at the top, by roughening or etching the surface or by placing retentive grooves
media	substance through which something else is introduced
median palatine suture	line of fusion of the two maxillae; runs between the maxillary central incisor and extends posterior across the palate
medical history	see health history
medicament	medicine that promotes healing from an injury or ailment
Medicare	federal insurance program that provides in-patient hospital services for all people over the age of 65 and to eligible disabled individuals

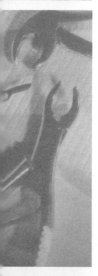

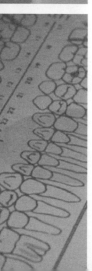

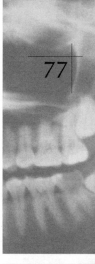

mental foramen	opening usually located between the apicies of the first and second mandibular premolars (bicuspids) for passage of blood vessels and nerves that supply the lips; viewed as a radiolucency on radiographs
mentalis muscle	muscle that moves the chin tissue and raises or lowers the lips
meperidine	narcotic used as an analgesic or sedative; generic name for Demerol®
mercury	dense liquid element (metal) that is mixed with a metal alloy to produce amalgam
mesial	surface of the tooth closest to the midline
mesiodens	a supernumerary tooth that usually appears between the maxillary central incisors; can be impacted or erupted
metabolize	to chemically change through the functions of nutrition; enables various substances (foods, drugs) to be used by the body
metastasize	to move; usually refers to malignant (cancerous) cells; movement of disease from one part of the body to another though blood vessels, lymph nodes or respiratory tract
methohexital sodium	short acting barbiturate injected intravenously prior to the use of general anesthetic because of its rapid induction of sleep; generic name for Brevital®
methylmethacrylate monomer	liquid catalyst mixed with a polymer to make a self-curing acrylic resin
methylmethacrylate polymer	powder mixed with a liquid catalyst (methylmethacrylate monomer) to make a self-curing resin
meticulous	concerned with details; very precise
microbes	see microorganism
microleakage	see page of saliva, debris and bacteria between the restoration and tooth structure
microorganism	microscopic living organism that may invade humans and create pathologic responses
midazolam	agent used for general and conscious sedation prior to performing some oral surgical procedures; generic name for Versed®
midline	imaginary vertical line between the mandibular and maxillary central incisors and running through the entire body dividing it into two equal halves

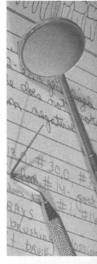

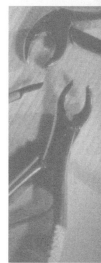

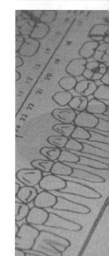

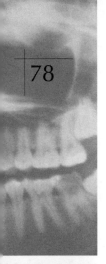
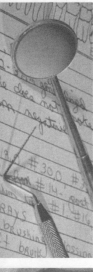
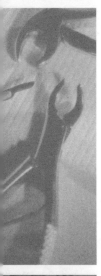
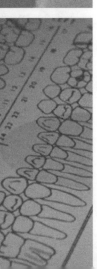

m

mid-sagittal	an imaginary vertical plane that equally separates the body into two halves; often referred to as the midline
milliamperage (mA)	measurement used to determine the amount of electrons emitted from a radiographic tubehead; increasing the milliamperage setting increases the amount of radiation emitted from the tubehead
minor treatment	includes restorations, equilibration, simple tooth removal, etc.
mitral valve	a two-flapped heart valve between the left atrium and left ventricle
mitral valve prolapse	condition of the mitral valve where one or both of the valve flaps are too large and balloon back into left atrium when ventricle contracts; valves may close and function normally or become dysfunctional allowing regurgitation of blood back into the atrium
mixed dentition	dentition consisting of a mixture of primary and permanent teeth; usually observed in children between the ages of 6 and 12
mobility	tooth movement caused by periodontal disease or trauma
model (laboratory) plaster	weak, very porous gypsum material used where strength or detail is not important
model trimmer	laboratory equipment (grinding device) used to trim or shape a variety of models made of gypsum products
molar	tooth located posterior to the premolars in each quadrant; purpose is to chew and grind food; maxillary first and second molars usually have trifurcated (3) roots and at least three canals; mandibular first and second molars usually have bifurcated (2) roots and at least two canals; the roots and canals on third molars vary in number
monomer	acrylic liquid; any molecule that can be bound to form a polymer
mononucleosis	communicable disease caused by a virus that affects the lymph tissues; is characterized by enlarged, tender lymph nodes, fever, a sore throat; an enlarged spleen and altered liver functions occurs in about half of patients
morphology	the study of anatomical form and structure
mortician	funeral director
mottled enamel	see fluorosis

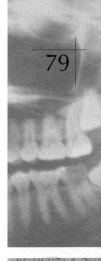

mouth guard	intraoral protective device worn to prevent the loss or fracture of teeth
mouth mirror	instrument used to see areas in the mouth that cannot be seen by direct vision or to reflect light or to retract the cheeks or tongue; used to protect the tissue from rotary cutting instruments
mouth prop	used to hold open a patient's mouth while under sedation or to reduce strain on jaw muscles
mouthwash	used for cleansing, germicidal and palliative properties
MPD	see maximum permissible dose
MRI	see magnetic resonance imaging
MSDS	see Material Safety Data Sheet
mucobuccal fold	muscle attachment of the oral mucous membrane as it passes from the mandible or maxilla to the cheek
mucocele	mucous or fluid filled cyst
mucogingival junction	line between the attached gingiva and the alveolar mucosa
mucoperiosteal flap	soft tissue that is incised and retracted from the bone
mucosa	moist tissue; lines the inner surface of the oral cavity, nasal passages and other moist anatomical area
mucous membrane	membrane that lines the oral cavity and is the first natural barrier that keeps bacteria from entering the body
mucus	fluid secreted by mucous membranes and salivary glands
mulberry molars	anomaly caused by congenital syphilis and involves all four first permanent molars; the occlusal surfaces of the molars appear more rounded, resembling a mulberry
murmur	abnormal sound heard in the region of the heart; can be caused by abnormalities of the heart valve, congenital abnormalities, heart infections, coronary artery disease or hypertension; may be an insignificant condition
muscle attachments	see frenum
mylar	heavy, cellophane-type material that provides matrix support for anterior areas

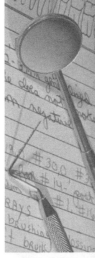

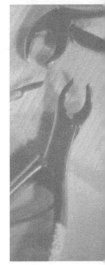

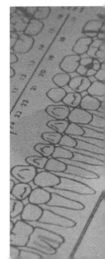

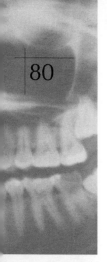

m

mylohyoid muscle	muscle that forms the floor of the mouth; elevates the tongue and lowers the jaw
mylohyoid ridge	line or ridge of bone located on the lingual side of the mandible and is the insertion point for the mylohyoid muscle
myocardial infarction	blockage of the arteries supplying the heart; heart attack

n

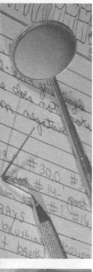

naloxone	drug used to counteract respiratory depression as a result of ingesting opiate narcotics; generic name for Narcan®
Narcan®	see naloxone
nasion	point where the middle of nasofrontal suture crosses the skull midplane
nasofrontal	relating to the frontal and nasal bones, nose and forehead
National Fire Protection Association's color and number method	labeling system for hazardous chemicals
nausea	queasy feeling in the stomach characterized by a feeling of the need to vomit
NCRP	acronym for National Council on Radiation Protection and Measurement
neck strap	device that attaches outside the oral cavity to orthodontic head-gear to supply stability and tension
necrosis	death of a cell or group of cells
necrotic	dead; often referred to in terms of dead tissue

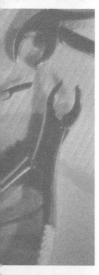

necrotizing ulcerative gingivitis	inflammation of the gingiva characterized by: necrosis of the interdental papillae, ulceration of the gingival margins, pain and foul odor; see acute necrotizing ulcerative gingivitis (ANUG)
needle	sharp-pointed hollow tube used to administer liquid agents intraorally, intravenously and intramuscularly; sharp instrument for suturing or passing ligature
needle holder	1) instrument similar to a hemostat but with a thicker, shorter beak used to hold a suture needle 2) safety devise used to hold a needle shaft for recapping
negligence	by an act of omission or commission doing something that a responsible person would not do

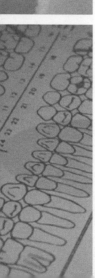

neoplasm	abnormal mass of tissue whose growth exceeds that of normal tissue; can be malignant or benign; tumor	*n*

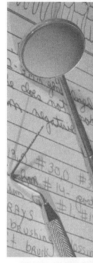

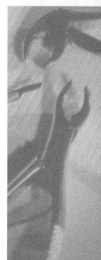

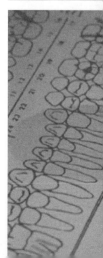

net income	accounts payable subtracted from the gross income
neural	connected to or related to the nervous system
neutralize	to render ineffective
nitrile gloves	latex-free gloves used in patient treatment, cleanup and instrument sterilization procedures
nitroglycerine	vasodilator used in the treatment of angina pectoris, taken sublingually or transdermally; i.e., a patch
nitroglycerine patch	patch that is affixed to the tissue that provides constant exposure to the medication
nitrous oxide	analgesic and sedative agent used in conjunction with oxygen to relieve anxiety and fear; administered by inhalation route
NNIS	acronym for national nosocomial infection systems
N$_2$O	chemical sign for nitrous oxide oxygen relative analgesia
noble metal	precious metal
NOCA	National Organization for CompetencyAssurance; see Appendix A
nodule	small node
noncorrosive	substance or instrument that will not corrode
nonpathogenic	unable to cause disease
nonsufficient funds (NSF)	bank checks returned to the office due to a lack of funds
normal sinus rhythm	term that indicates the heart is operating within normal parameters; heart beat is normal
nosocomial	disease arising in a hospital or other healthcare settings; i.e., staph infection
NSF	see nonsufficient funds

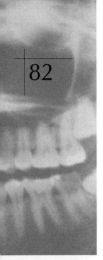
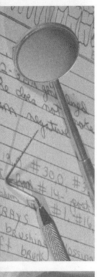
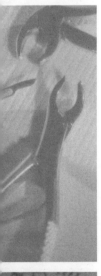
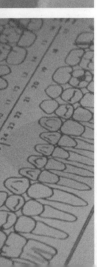

n

nuclear magnetic resonance — procedure where the body is filled with small biological magnets (the most abundant and responsive is the proton) and placed into an MRI facility (see magnetic resonance imaging) which creates a steady state within the body by placing the body in a steady magnetic field and stimulates the body with radio waves to change the steady-state orientation of protons; it then stops the radio waves and listens to the body's electromagnetic transmissions at a selected frequency; the transmitted signal is used to construct internal images of the body

nullify — to make invalid

nursing bottle syndrome — gross amounts of decay in the teeth of children caused by ingestion of liquids containing sugars, often placed in bottles and given to infants at bed time

nystagmus — involuntary, irregular movement of the eyes in a circular movement in any direction

o

O_2 — chemical sign for oxygen

obturate — to fill; often used when discussing filling a root canal

occlude — to close together the maxillary and mandibular teeth

occlusal — the top or chewing surface of the premolars and molars

occlusal equilibration — adjusting of occlusal surfaces of teeth to remove all interferences on the teeth

occlusal film — radiograph taken to obtain a wider view of the maxilla or mandible on a single film

occlusal pits — small point in the occlusal surface of enamel located at either end of a developmental groove or where two grooves cross or meet

occlusal plane — imaginary surface that touches the incisal edges of the incisors and the cusp tips of the posterior teeth

occlusal registration — see bite registration

occupational exposure — reasonably anticipated skin, eye, mucous membrane or parenteral contact with blood or OPIM that can result from the performance of an employee's duties

odontectomy — extraction of a tooth

odontoblasts — dentin-forming cells

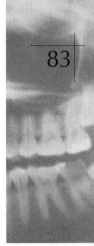

OFD	acronym for object to film distance
OHI	acronym for oral hygiene instruction
one handed scoop technique	safety technique employed to recap needles without touching the needle; used when some form of safety device is not available
onlay	gold or porcelain restoration that covers one or more cusps, but not all cusps of a tooth
operator	person performing dentistry on a patient: dentist, hygienist, registered or expanded function dental assistant
OPIM	acronym for other potentially infectious materials
opposing dentition	teeth that are opposite each other, i.e., maxillary teeth over the mandibular teeth
optimum level	the amount or degree of something that is most favorable to some end; such as when fluoride content of the teeth is increased to a level that is likely reduce the effects of the caries process
oral and maxillofacial pathology	specialty of dentistry and discipline of pathology that deals with the nature, identification and management of diseases affecting the oral and maxillofacial regions; a science that investigates the causes, processes and effects of these diseases; and includes research and diagnosis of diseases using clinical, radiographic, microscopic, biochemical or other examinations
oral and maxillofacial radiology	specialty of dentistry and discipline of radiology concerned with the production and interpretation of images and data produced by all modalities of radiant energy that are used for the diagnosis and management of diseases, disorders and conditions of the oral and maxillofacial region
oral and maxillofacial surgery	specialty of dentistry that includes the diagnosis, surgical and adjunctive treatment of diseases, injuries and defects involving both the functional and esthetic aspects of the hard and soft tissues of the oral and maxillofacial region
oral cavity	the mouth
oral pathology	dental specialty that involves the diagnosis and nature of diseases that effect the oral cavity
orange solvent	substance used to remove temporary cement and for other cleaning purposes
organic matter	carbon based material

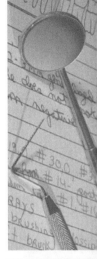

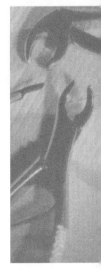

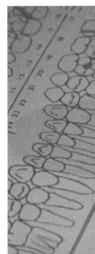

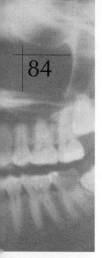

O

orthodontic band	thin band of stainless steel placed on posterior teeth to which brackets are soldered for the attachment of an arch wire
orthodontic protractor	triangular shaped form used to make cephalometric tracings
orthodontics	dental specialty that diagnoses and corrects abnormally aligned dentitions
orthodontics and dentofacial orthopedics	area of dentistry concerned with the supervision, guidance and correction of the growing or mature dentofacial structures, including those conditions that require movement of teeth or correction of malrelationships and malformations of their related structures and the adjustment of relationships between and among teeth and facial bones by the application of forces and/or the stimulation and redirection of functional forces within the craniofacial complex; major responsibilities of orthodontic practice include the diagnosis, prevention, interception and treatment of all forms of malocclusion of the teeth and associated alterations in their surrounding structures; the design, application and control of functional and corrective appliances: and the guidance of the dentition and its supporting structures to attain and maintain optimum occlusal relations in physiologic and esthetic harmony among facial and cranial structures
orthodontic scaler	instrument used to direct brackets for placement, remove elastics and cement and/or bonding material
orthodontic stone	mixture of model plaster and laboratory stone used to fabricate models
orthodontist	dental specialist that diagnoses and treats malaligned teeth
orthognathic surgery	surgery involving the face, maxilla and mandible; usually part of orthodontic treatment
OSAP	Organization for Safety and Asepsis Procedures; see Appendix A
OSHA	Occupational Safety and Health Administration; see Appendix A
OSHA Bloodborne Pathogens Standard	national standard that defines what employers must do to protect workers against occupational exposure to bloodborne pathogens
OSHA Hazard Communication Standard	see Hazard Communication Standard
osseointegration	uniting of bone and an implant
osseous	related to the bone

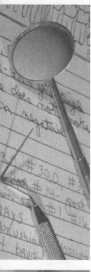

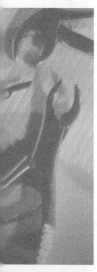

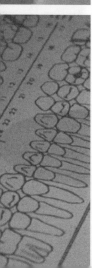

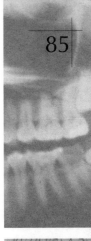

osseous surgery	surgery performed to repair defects or deformities in the bone caused by periodontal disease and other conditions
osteitis	inflammation of the bone; characterized by tenderness and dull, aching pain
osteoblasts	cells that form bone; associated with growth and development
osteoclasts	cells responsible for resorption and remodeling of the bone
osteoplasty	surgical procedure performed to reshape bone
osteoporosis	a condition that is seen as a loss of bone mass with decreased density and enlargement of bone spaces resulting in more porosity and fragility
osteotomy	surgical procedure for removal of bone
OTC	acronym for over-the-counter
outstanding balance	amount of money owed to the dental practice
outstanding check	check that has not been cashed and has not been subtracted from the account by the bank
overdenture	denture placed over retained roots that may contain posts and cores with attachments in a full or partial denture to supply support
overexpose	radiographic film that is too dark; caused by incorrect exposure settings
over-exposure	unnecessary exposure to radiation
overhang	excess amalgam or composite beyond the margin of a cavity preparation
overlapping	radiographic error caused by incorrect horizontal angulation creating the inability to see the mesial and/or distal surfaces of the exposed teeth
oxygen	element required for breathing; used in conjunction with nitrous oxide to maintain an adequate level of oxygen in the body in medical emergencies where respiratory difficulty is evident
oxygenating rinse	agent fused with oxygen that has a bubbling action when used

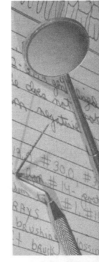

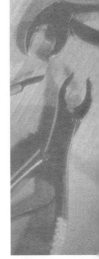

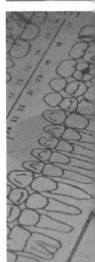

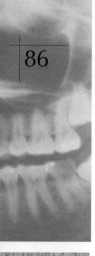
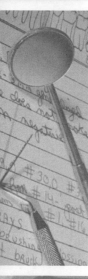
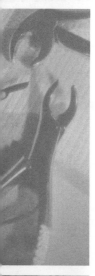
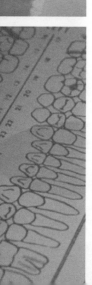

p

PA	acronym for periapical radiographs; see periapical
packing cord	see retraction cord
packing slip	list of supplies enclosed in a shipment
palatal	pertaining to the palate; term often used when referring the lingual, or tongue side of maxillary teeth
palatal separating appliance	screw-like orthodontic device used to expand the mid-palatal suture
palatal vault	1) height of the palatal portion of a denture 2) curved shape of the bones that form the palate
palate	bone and soft tissue that forms the roof of the mouth
palliative	temporary treatment given to relieve pain
palpation	extraoral examination procedure used to check the consistency of tissue; examining soft tissue by gently squeezing between the fingers
pancreatitis	inflammation of the pancreas that presents with symptoms of intense pain, vomiting, belching and sometimes hiccoughing
panoramic radiograph	extraoral radiograph taken to expose the maxillary and mandibular arches, tempormandibular joints and associated anatomy on a single film
paper pad	stack of paper on which various dental materials are mixed
paper point	cone of absorbent paper used to dry canals in an endodontic procedure, to place medication in a canal, or to inoculate cultures
papillae	any small, pointed elevation (note: papilla is the singular form of the word, papillae is the plural form)

Types

circumvallate papillae (or vallate papillae)–	8-12 mushroom shaped papillae that form a "V" at the sulcus terminalis which divides the body of the tongue (anterior 2/3) from the root (posterior 1/3)
filiform papillae–	finger-like projections that cover the dorsal surface of the tongue and provides the sense of touch

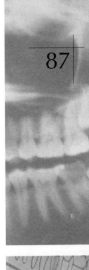

papillae *(continued)* | fungiform papillae– | dark red, small, flat papilla scattered throughout the middle and anterior dorsal surface and the sides of the tongue which house a few taste buds and specialize in sweet taste

p

papilloma — a benign neoplasm of epithelium often having a warty appearance; a benign, peduculated, cauliflower-like neoplasm of epithelium

parallel — two lines or planes at equal distance at all points

paralleling technique — radiographic technique where the film is placed parallel to the long axis of the tooth and the central x-ray beam is at a right angle to the teeth and film

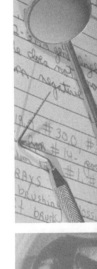

parenteral transmission — infection contracted through the skin and can be associated with injections or oral piercing

paresthesia —
1) an altered sensation reported by the patient in an area where the sensory nerve has been afflicted by a disease or an injury;
2) loss of sensation, burning, or prickling of the lip, tongue and teeth caused by cutting or nicking a nerve

Parkinson's disease — chronic, progressive, debilitating disease of the nervous system that presents with fine, slow tremors, muscular weakness and rigidity

parotid gland — largest of the salivary glands; positioned at the side of the face just below and in front of the ear along the posterior border of the ramus of the mandible; produces serous fluid

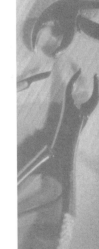

partially erupted — tooth that has not fully erupted into the dentition

participating dentist — a dentist that has an agreement to render care to subscribers under rules and regulations of a particular insurance plan

particulate — formed of separate particles

partnership — legal association or contract defining the association of two or more persons in a business or professional relationship

pathogenic — causing disease

pathogens — disease producing microorganisms

patient napkin — napkin that is placed over the patient to protect his or her clothing during treatment

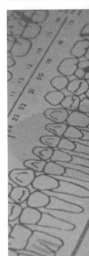

patient record — consists of the medical and dental history of a patient

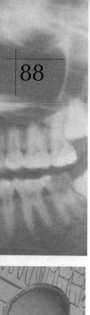
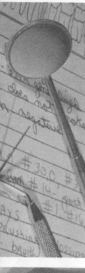
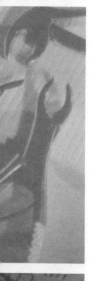
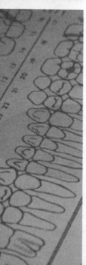

p

PDR	acronym for Physician's Desk Reference
pediatric dentist	practitioner that specializes in treating children
pediatric dentistry	age-defined specialty that provides both primary and comprehensive preventive and therapeutic oral health care for infants and children through adolescence, including those with special health care needs
pedicle flap	performed to replace tissue lost from recession on a single tooth: a flap of tissue is made with lateral incisions partially cut away with one edge still attached, then the flap is slid sideways to cover the exposed root and sutured in place
pedunculated	being attached to or growing on; having a stalk; such as a tissue tag
pellicle	thin, clear film or membrane of insoluble proteins, fats and other materials from saliva that reforms within minutes of removal and harbors bacterial pathogens
penetrate	to enter into or infiltrate
penicillin	antibiotic used to prevent and treat infections
penumbra	term applied to the fuzzy or unclear area that surrounds all radiographic images; the amount of penumbra can be reduced by reducing the size of the focal spot on the target of the x-ray anode
PEP	acronym for post exposure prophylaxis
percolate	to seep through as in water through coffee grounds 1) removal of the soluble parts of a drug by slowly allowing a liquid solvent to flow through it 2) an undesirable (negative) effect of fluid movement between the restorative material and tooth structure during times of expansion and contraction that occurs with most restorative materials; can result in possible irritation to the dental pulp and recurrent decay
percutaneous	through the skin; occupational exposure of pathogens introduced though the skin with a needle or instrument
perforate	to pierce or punch a hole
periapical	pertaining to around the apex; radiograph that exposes the entire tooth and surrounding tissues
periapical abscess	accumulation of exudate located at the apex of a tooth causing an infection

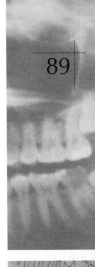

pericoronitis	inflammation of the tissues around the crown of a tooth, typically with erupting third molars
periodontal disease	inflammation and deterioration of the periodontal tissues that causes loss of gingival attachment due to tissue resorption
periodontal dressing	non-eugenol or zinc oxide eugenol based surgical dressing placed over the tissues and around the necks of teeth to protect the site after surgery
periodontal fibers (ligament)	connective tissue that supports and suspends the teeth in position with fibers that attach to the alveolar process or cementum

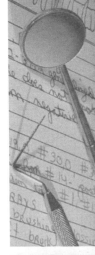

Types

alveolar crest fibers–	retains the tooth in the socket and opposes lateral forces
apical fibers–	prevents the tooth from tipping, resists luxation and protects the blood, lymph and nerve supplies
horizontal fibers–	restrains lateral tooth movement
interradicular fibers–	aids in resisting tipping and twisting of the tooth
oblique fibers–	resists forces placed on the long axis of the tooth

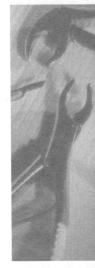

periodontal flap surgery	procedure performed to separate the gingiva from the teeth and bone to enable procedures such as scaling and root planning and recontouring of the underlying bone
periodontal pocket	sulcus depth that is greater than 3mm
periodontal probe	instrument with calibrated marks used to measure the depth of periodontal pockets
periodontics	specialty of dentistry which encompasses the prevention, diagnosis and treatment of diseases of the supporting and surrounding tissues of the teeth or their substitutes and the maintenance of the health, function and esthetics of these structures and tissues
periodontist	practitioner that diagnoses and treats diseases of the periodontal tissues
periodontitis	bacterial infection characterized by inflammation of the gingiva and supporting tissues with pocket formation and bone loss
periodontium	supporting tissues of the teeth; i.e., gingiva, cementum, periodontal ligament, and alveolar bone

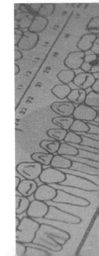

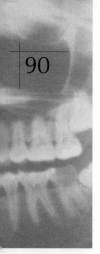
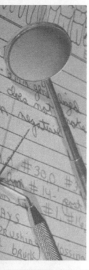
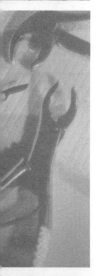
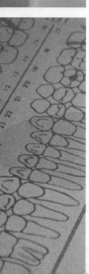

p

periodontosis	rare disease, without a recognizable cause, found in young people, primarily in women; symptoms include: swelling, bleeding gums, and retraction of gums with a significant loss of soft tissue and bone
periosteal elevator	instrument used to retract tissue from the bone; see elevator
periosteum	fibrous connective tissue covering bones in the oral cavity that contains blood, lymph vessels, osteoblasts and nerve tissue
periphery	outer edge or border of something
periradicular	around the root
permanent dentition (teeth)	32 teeth that erupt as, or after the primary dentition (teeth) have been shed
pernicious anemia	blood disease that causes muscular weakness, gastrointestinal and neural disturbances
perpendicular	two lines or planes intersecting at right angles
personal protective equipment (PPE)	equipment worn by a health care worker that provides protection against contamination from microorganisms
personal supervision	see supervision
petty cash	small amount of cash in an office available for small purchases
pH	measure of acidity or alkalinity of a solution
pharynx	passageway for air from the nasal cavity to the larynx and food from the mouth to the esophagus
phenolics	liquids used for intermediate-level disinfection
phenytoin	anticonvulsant that is used in the treatment of epilepsy; generic name for Dilantin®
PHI	acronym for protected health information
phosphor	crystalline substance that covers intensifying screens and emits visible light when exposed to x-rays
phosphoric acid	see etchant
Physician's Desk Reference (PDR)	publication that defines uses and contraindications for drugs
PID	see position indicating device
pigmented	coloration of tissues caused by an organic deposit in the body that contains color (melanin)

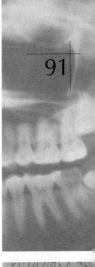

pin and ligature cutter	instrument used to cut the ligature wire after placement and in the removal of the archwire; used to cut retention pins
pin retention	strengthening a core build-up or large restoration by use of pins
pit and fissure sealant	resin material placed on the occlusal surfaces of premolars and molars to fill in deep grooves and crevices; applied to prevent the formation of decay
plaque	sticky substance that accumulates on the surfaces of the teeth; derived from saliva and bacteria and their products; is a factor in tooth decay and gingival inflammation
plaster	gypsum-based material used primarily to mount casts to an articulator
platelets	small, irregular, colorless cells that are formed in the red bone marrow; important in forming clots
plugger	instrument to compress restorative material in the cavity preparation
polish	to make smooth and glossy
polishing brush	brush used to polish the occlusal surfaces of teeth to clean deep pits and fissures, restorations, and removable appliances
polishing cup	flexible rubber cup used to polish teeth and appliances
polycarboxylate cement	permanent cement used for seating (cementing) crowns, bridges, inlays, onlays, orthodontic bands and brackets; does not create exothermic heat when curing
polyether	impression material used for the fabrication of crowns and bridges
polymer	a synthetic substance made of two or more molecules
polymerization	see curing
polyvinyl siloxane	highly accurate, tear resistant, stable impression material used for crown and bridge procedures
pontic	artificial tooth that replaces a missing tooth in a fixed bridge or removable appliance
porcelain	hard ceramic material used in the fabrication of crowns, inlays, onlays and veneers
porosity	having pores or voids in a substance

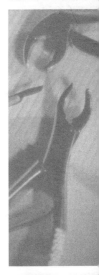

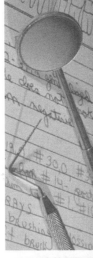

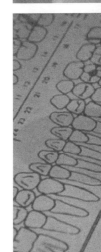

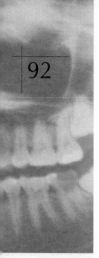

p

position indicating device (PID)	lead-lined cylindrical or rectangular open-ended portion of the tubehead that emits radiation
post dam	posterior edge of a denture that helps maintain suction to hold the denture into place
posterior	to the back; refers to the premolars and molars in the permanent dentition and molars in the primary dentition
posterior band remover	instrument with a cushioned tip used to remove orthodontic bands from posterior teeth
Postexposure Management Program	clearly defined policies, procedures and education of dental healthcare personnel (DHCP) in the rapid access to clinical care, Post Exposure Prophylaxis (PEP) and testing sources
post-operative instructions	directions given to a patient after a surgical or restorative procedure to ensure proper healing and patient comfort
potassium sulfate	material used to increase the setting time of gypsum products
potentiate	to increase effectiveness of a drug, often by supplementing with another drug
povidone iodine	liquid used to destroy a variety of microorganisms, clean wounds, and disinfect for preoperative tissue preparation; generic name for Betadine®
PPE	see personal protection equipment
ppm	acronym for parts per million
PPO	see Preferred Provider Organization
precise	exact; accurate
predispose	inclined to do
prefabricated	constructed in advance
Preferred Provider Organization (PPO)	organization that pays a fixed price to a designated provider (dentist) for providing specified services to those who have benefits
preliminary inspection	an initial or first examination or inspection of the oral cavity and facial structures
premedication	medication given to a patient prior to treatment, often an antibiotic or sedative
premolar	tooth located between the canines and molars in each quadrant; purpose is to pulverize food; first premolars have a bifurcated root and two canals, second premolars have one root and one canal; sometimes referred to as bicuspids

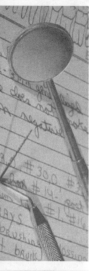

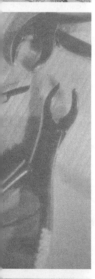

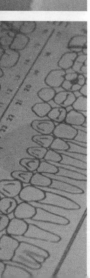

p

pre-operative instructions	instructions given to a patient before a surgical or restorative procedure
preset trays	trays prepared ahead of time with all instruments and supplies required for a specific procedure
pressure gauge	instrument that shows the level of pressure attained
pressure pot	piece of equipment similar to a pressure cooker that is used to harden acrylic for oral appliances
preventive treatment	treatment provided to prevent disease, including prophylaxis, fluoride treatments, etc.; treatment provided to arrest a degenerative condition
primary beam	see central ray
primary carrier	insurance plan covering the patient who is the employee or the plan that covers a dependent in accordance with the birthday rule
primary dentition	20 teeth that are replaced by the permanent dentition
prion diseases	fatal degenerative diseases of the central nervous system that occur when normal forms of proteins on cell surfaces of the central nervous system (CNS) and lymphoreticular tissues mutate into an infectious form that changes how they react with other brain chemicals
prn	abbreviation that indicates a patient is to take the prescribed medication as needed
process indicator	a variety of different modalities that allow for visual verification that a package of dental instruments has been exposed to in the sterilization process; shows that physical and/or chemical conditions necessary for sterilization have been achieved but does not indicate that sterilization has occurred
processing solutions	see developer and fixer
prochlorperazine	drug administered to counteract nausea; generic name for Compazine®
prognathic	anatomical configuration in which the upper and lower jaws protrude beyond the forehead
promiscuous	indiscriminate; casual; random
prone	lying with face down
prophylactic antibiotics	antibiotics taken prior to an invasive procedure to prevent infection

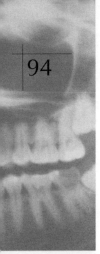

p

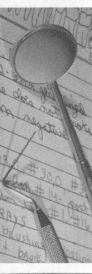

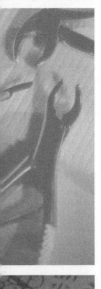

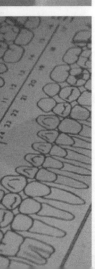

prophylaxis	procedure performed to remove calculus and polish teeth with a polishing cup and mild abrasive
prophylaxis angle	see handpieces
prophylaxis paste	agent used to polish teeth
prosthesis	artificial replacement of one or more missing teeth or tooth structure(s); or for a missing limb or other body part
prosthodontics	branch of dentistry pertaining to the restoration and maintenance of oral functions, comfort, appearance and health of the patient by the restoration of natural teeth and/or the replacement of missing teeth and contiguous oral and maxillofacial tissues with artificial substitutes
protective eyewear	goggles or glasses with shields worn by health care providers and patients to protect the wearer from injury or infection from spray or spatter or flying objects
protected health information (PHI)	personal information, defined by the Health Insurance Portability & Accountability Act (HIPAA), that would identify a patient
prothrombin time	test performed to determine the first stage of blood coagulation
protrude	to jut out or project
provider	the dentist, or whomever renders professional service, as related to insurance terminology
proximal	mesial or distal surface of the tooth that is nearest the adjacent tooth
proximity	being near or next to
provisional restoration	temporary filling for a cavity preparation or covering for a crown and/or bridge preparation
pruritis	allergic reaction, resulting in itching, caused from hives releasing histamine from cells in the skin ; with a severe reaction, the face and throat may swell causing problems with breathing, creating the danger of suffocation
psi	acronym for pounds per square inch
pterygoid muscle	muscle of mastication that elevates the mandible
pulmonary edema	congestion of the veins associated with congestive heart failure; swelling due to fluid build-up tends to appear first in the feet and legs, and then move up the body

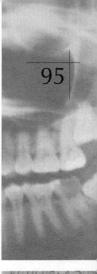

pulp	tissue found in the center of the tooth and made of blood vessels, lymph tissue and nerves; responsible for tactile sensations
pulp canal	portion of the pulp that is found in the root section of the tooth
pulp capping	covering exposed pulp for protection

Types
indirect–	placement of calcium hydroxide to promote healing when decay is removed that is very close to the pulp, but has not been exposed
direct–	placement of calcium hydroxide to provide a protective base over a slight pulp exposure

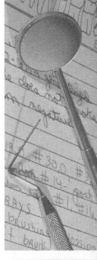

pulp chamber	large portion of the pulp that is located in the crown of the tooth
pulp horns	extensions of the pulp that project toward the cusp tips and incisal edges of the tooth
pulp stones	calcification found in the pulp chamber of a tooth
pulp test	test performed to determine the vitality of a tooth; includes heat, cold, electrical, percussion and others
pulpectomy	root canal treatment which involves complete removal of the pulp and filling the canal with gutta-percha
pulpitis	inflammation of the pulp
pulpotomy	partial removal of the pulp which is typically done in primary teeth

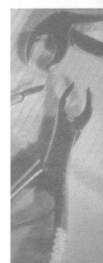

pumice	volcanic ash material used to polish teeth, removable and provisional restorations
puncture resistant container	rigid plastic container for depositing sharps
puncture wound	hole made in skin from penetration of a sharp object
purge	to cleanse or purify; to rid or empty of impurities
purulent discharge	pus
pus	an inflammatory exudate or discharge; usually bacterial
pyogenic granuloma	a hyperplastic lesion that appears as a red, rounded, painless growth of tissue that extends from the surface of the mucosa; often called pregnancy tumor; is found in males and non-pregnant females

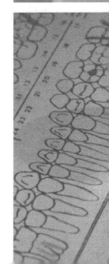

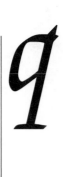

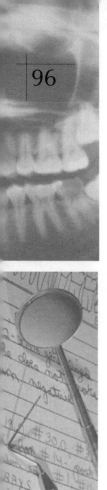

q

QC	acronym for quality control
qid	indicates the patient is to take the prescribed medication four times a day
quadrant	portion of the dentition comprised of a central incisor through third molar; there are four quadrants in the oral cavity
quick connect	coupling used to attach a handpiece to a hose with a simple movement

r

rad	see radiation absorbed dose
radial artery	artery on the inner surface of the wrist used for taking a pulse
radiation	process of emission, transmission and absorption of radiant energy

<u>Types</u>

gamma–	photons that have a shorter wavelength than used in diagnostic dental radiography
ionizing–	process by which electrons are removed from an atom resulting in an ion pair; a negatively charged free electron and the remaining part of the atom, now positively charged; waves contain energy sufficient to overcome the binding energy of electrons in atoms or molecules, creating ions; includes x-rays and gamma rays; can cause cell death in high doses over a short period of time, and errors in the reproductive process (mutations) in lower doses over longer periods of time
primary–	all radiation produced directly from the target in an x-ray tube
scattered–	radiation that has been deflected from its path; may include secondary radiation
secondary–	created by primary radiation when it comes into contact with matter such as the face and head

radiation absorbed dose (rad)	amount of energy absorbed per unit mass of tissue at a determined site
radiation exposure	amount of radiation a person is exposed to at a particular time

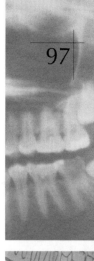

radiation hygiene	science of protection against injury by radiation
radiograph	image produced on a radiation-sensitive film emulsion by exposing the film to radiation and chemicals so that a negative is produced
radiographic mount	plastic or cardboard material in which radiographs are arranged to correspond with the location of their images in the oral cavity
radiography	process of taking radiographs
radiolucent	producing dark images on a film because a large amount of radiation interacts with the film; refers to structures that are easily penetrated by x-rays; i.e., pulp, bone, foramen
radiopaque	producing light images on film because only a small amount of radiation interacts with the film; refers to structures that absorb radiation; i.e., amalgam, gutta percha
rag wheel	device used on a lathe to polish appliances
raised dots	raised protrusions on radiographs used to orient radiographs to determine where specific periapical and bitewing radiographs are to be placed in a mount
ramus of the mandible	portion of the mandible that extends upward and backwards from the horseshoe-shaped body and terminates in two processes
ranula	mucus-containing space located in the floor of the mouth created from an obstruction of the ducts and sublingual salivary glands
rbc	acronym for red blood cells
RCT	acronym for root canal therapy; see root canal
recall appointment	preventive care appointment made at a pre-determined interval appropriate to fulfill a patient's dental health care needs
recare appointment	see recall appointment
recare system	integral part of a practice where patients are informed when they are due for a recare/recall appointment
receipts	money collected from patients and other debtors
recession	decline or reduction in the height of the gingival tissues which can include resorption of the alveolar crest; loss of tissue by apical migration
records management	maintenance of patient and financial records and protection against their loss or damage

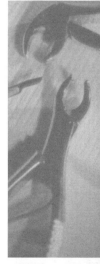

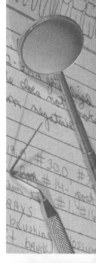

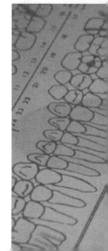

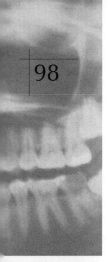

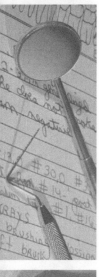

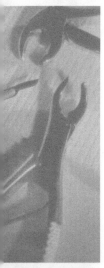

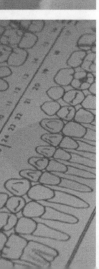

r

recurrent	repeating
referral slip	written form completed by the dentist referring a patient to a specialist
regenerate	to form new tissue
regulated waste	potentially infectious materials or items that could cause harm; types of waste that are regulated by the Environmental Protection Agency and each state
regurgitate	to throw up
rehabilitation	to restore to a useful condition
release of information	statement on an insurance form signed by the insured which allows the dentist to provide to an insurance carrier information pertaining to that patient's treatment; form completed by the patient allowing release of information to another medical professional
Rem	acronym for radiation equipment man
remineralization	process of restoring lost mineral salts to tissues such as bone, enamel, dentin or cementum
removable partial denture	prosthesis that replaces one or more, but not all teeth and is able to be removed
reorder point	point at which a specific item must be re-ordered to avoid running out
replenish	to re-fill; to make whole
reposition	to move into a different area or position
reservoir bag	bag attached to a nitrous oxide machine in which the nitrous oxide and oxygen are mixed and from which the patient takes in the gas
residual	left over
resin	cement used as luting agent or for cementation of orthodontic bands
resorption	horizontal or vertical bone or tissue loss caused from periodontal disease
respiration	process of breathing
respiratory obstruction	foreign material or object lodged in the airway that obstructs breathing
restoration	amalgam or composite filling, crown or inlay
restrict	constrain; limit

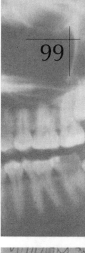

resuscitation mask (one way valve)	plastic apparatus placed over a victim's mouth and nose through which the rescuer breaths to administer oxygen; prevents contamination from body fluids between the victim and rescuer
retainer	custom made appliance used to retain the teeth in their positions after the fixed appliances have been removed

Types
1) **Biteplane**
2) **Cervical headgear**
3) **Functional**
4) **Frankel**
5) **Herbst**
6) **Palatal expander**
7) **Positioner**
8) **Retainer**
9) **Space maintainer**

retention	mechanical or chemical securing of a restoration
retraction cord (packing cord)	cord placed around the tooth to widen the sulcus to allow impression material to flow beyond the margin of the preparation

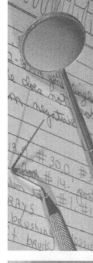

Types
impregnated– contains an astrigent-vasoconstrictor chemical to help control bleeding and shrink tissues

nonimpregnated– does not contain any chemicals and retracts tissues by a mechanical method

retrognathic	anatomical configuration in which the lower jaw is positioned posterior in relationship to other facial structures
retrograde	restoration placed at the apex of a tooth when the seal from an endodontic treatment is not satisfactory
retromolar pad	soft tissue posterior to the last molar in the mandible on each side

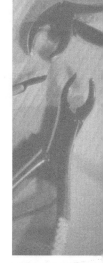

reversible hydrocolloid	impression material that can change from a solid or gel to a liquid form and back again
rheumatic fever	bacterial disease characterized by upper respiratory tract inflammation, lymph node involvement, arthritis and cardiac involvement, among other signs and symptoms
rheumatoid arthritis	chronic disease characterized by inflammation of the joints, stiffness, swelling and increase in the size of the cartilage and pain

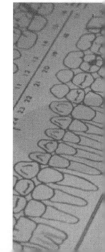

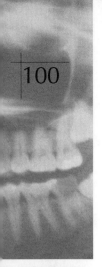

r

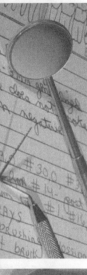

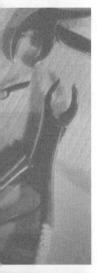

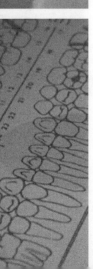

RHS	acronym for the national DANB Radiation Health & Safety component exam
rickets	disease caused by a deficiency in vitamin D that can result in an inadequate intake or excessive loss of calcium causing abnormalities in shape and structure of bone
rigid	very stiff; does not bend
rongeurs	instrument used to trim sharp projections on the alveolar bone after multiple extractions and to shape the edentulous ridge
root	part of the human tooth that is composed primarily of dentin and covered by cementum
root canal	1) canal located in the root(s) of the teeth which houses the pulp 2) treatment which involves the extirpation (removal) of diseased pulp tissues and filling of the empty canal
root caries	decay at or apical to the cementoenamel junction
root fragments	pieces of a tooth left in the socket after removal
root planing	smoothing of the surface of the roots of the teeth after removal of calculus and plaque
root resorption	shortening or narrowing of the root of a tooth due to trauma
root tip pick	instrument used to remove root tips or fragments in a socket
rotary cutting instruments (burs)	small cutters used in slow- and high-speed handpieces to cut tooth structure and bone or for finishing acrylic material

Bur materials

Carbide burs– rotary cutting instrument made of steel or tungsten; cutting burs usually have 8-12 flutes (cutting edges) while finishing burs have up to 40 flutes

Diamond burs– rotary cutting instruments with diamond particles imbedded in the bur head

Types/shapes of Carbide Burs

round– removes carious tooth structure

inverted cone– removes carious tooth structure to place retention grooves or undercuts in a preparation

plain fissure straight– forms walls of the preparation and places retention grooves

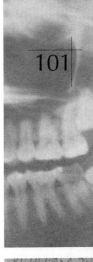

plain fissure cross-cut–	forms walls of the preparation and places retention grooves; has horizontal cross cuts
tapered fissure straight bur–	forms divergent wall of the preparation
tapered fissure cross cut–	forms divergent wall of the preparation; has horizontal cross cuts
end cutting–	cutting portion is on the end of the bur
Gates-Glidden–	football shaped bur used in a low-speed handpiece to enlarge the top portion of a canal during an endodontic procedure
pear–	opens and extends the preparation

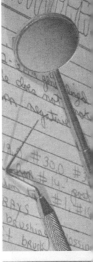

Types of Diamond Burs

prestressed–	fastest cutting; used for bulk removal of tooth structure
micrograin–	medium-fast cutting; used for controlled cutting and contouring
finisher–	fine grain; used to refine and smooth marginal areas, remove line angles and to finish subgingivally
superfinisher–	finest grain; used to contour and finish composite materials
round end taper–	used to remove tooth structure; for crown preparation and to make retention grooves
flat end taper–	makes square shoulders for crown preparations
cylinder–	smoothes and finishes walls where parallel sides and flat floors are needed
flame–	makes subgingival bevels in crown preparations
round–	used to access the pulp chamber; adjusts occlusal surfaces; reduces the lingual surfaces of anterior teeth
wheel–	prepares anterior crowns and shapes occlusal surfaces

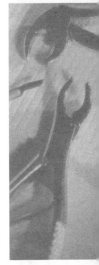

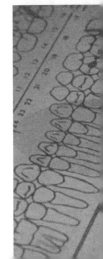

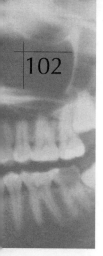

r

rotation	orthodontically moving a tooth in a desired direction
rouge	polishing agent for gold
rubber bowl	flexible bowl used to mix alginate or other materials
rubber dam	see dental dam
rubber points	flexible attachment impregnated with a polishing agent; used to polish anatomic grooves of metallic restorations
rubber stops	small, round pieces of rubber or plastic that are placed at a predetermined length on an endodontic file to prevent the file from perforating the apex of a tooth
Rx	acronym for prescription

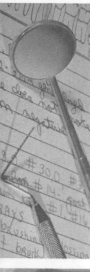

s

safelight	light used in a darkroom that will not cause fogging of the radiographic film
safety officer	dental health personnel (DHCP) assigned the responsibility of managing office safety and compliance with the Occupational Safety and Health Administration (OSHA)standards; see infection control officer (ICO)
sagittal	an imaginary plane that separates the body vertically but does not have to be into equal halves
saline solution	salt solution used as a rinse during surgical procedures
saliva	fluid secreted by glands in the oral cavity that has cleansing, lubricating, bacteriocidal and digestive functions
saliva ejector	disposable evacuation tip that is small in diameter and used to remove fluids from the oral cavity
sandpaper strip	long, narrow strip of material with an abrasive surface used to smooth interproximal surfaces
sanitize	to make clean
SARS	acronym for severe acute respiratory syndrome
saturated	when a porous substance is soaked by a liquid to its maximum capacity
SBE	see subacute bacterial endocarditis

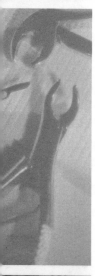

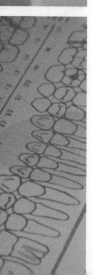

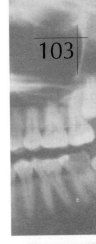

scaler	instrument used to remove plaque, calculus and stain
scaling	process of removing plaque, calculus and stain
scalpel	surgical knife used to cut or excise tissue
scarlet fever	contagious disease that presents with a sore throat, strawberry tongue, fever, scarlet rash and rapid pulse
scattered radiation	radiation whose direction has been redirected; also known as secondary radiation
scavenger system	safety system that reduces the amount of nitrous oxide gas released into the atmosphere
scribe	to write, trace or mark by making a line or lines with a pointed instrument or carbon marker
sealant	see pit and fissure sealant
secondary carrier	plan covering the patient as a dependent when the patient is the spouse or dependent child of a parent whose birthday occurs later in the calendar year
secondary container	container other than the original that a chemical is transferred into
secondary dentin	material that forms on the walls of the pulp chambers and canals after tooth eruption and continues to form at an extremely slow rate throughout the life of the tooth
secondary radiation	see scattered radiation
sedative	medication that has a tranquilizing effect
seizure	convulsion; interruption of motor and sensory functions due to an injury to the nervous system
self cure	see curing
sensitivity	tooth easily irritated from percussion, temperature, sweets, etc.
separator	device used to slightly separate the teeth to allow for the placement of orthodontic bands
serial extraction	interceptive orthodontic method employed to correct excessive overcrowding of the teeth in a single arch
seroconversion	the change of a serological test (blood test to detect the presence of antibodies against a microorganism) from negative (microorganism is not present) to positive (microorganism is present)
serous fluid	thick fluid with the color and viscosity of serum

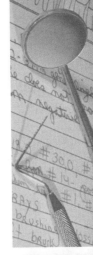

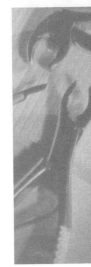

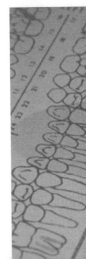

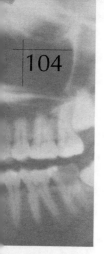

S

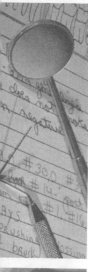

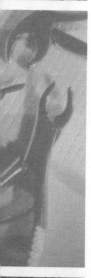

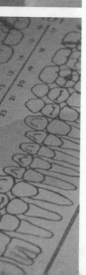

serum — clear, yellowish fluid obtained when blood is separated into its solid and liquid components after clotting

setting time — length of time it takes for a material to completely cure from the start of the mix process to hardening

shade guide — device containing a variety of shades used to match the natural shade of a tooth

shank — stem on which the working portion of a bur is attached

Type of Bur Shanks

long straight– designed for use in a low-speed handpiece (HP)

latch type– has a notch on the end that fits into a contra-angle/right angle handpiece (RA)

friction grip– short, small shank used in friction grip high-speed handpieces (FG)

sharpness — in radiology, the ability to reproduce a distinct outline of an object; also known as resolution or definition

sharps — items, including but not limited to, needles, scalpel blades, broken glass and orthodontic wires that can cut, stick or puncture which are disposed of according to the Occupational Safety and Health Administration's (OSHA's) Bloodborne Pathogens Standards

shear — to cut

shelf life — predetermined amount of time before a product begins to break down or deteriorate

shock — state of body collapse which leads to slowing of blood flow to the extremities and reduced cardiac output; disturbance of function, equilibrium or mental faculties from a drug reaction, trauma, hemorrhage, dehydration, etc.

sialoangiitis — inflammation of salivary gland ducts

sialogogue — substance that increases salivary flow

sialography — radiograph taken after the injection of a radiopaque material into the affected salivary gland; the main salivary glands studied with this radiograph are the parotid, submandibular and sublingual glands

sigmoid notch — forms the upper boarder of the ramus between the condyle and coronoid process

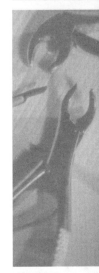

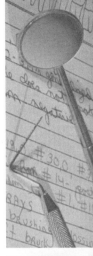

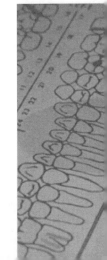

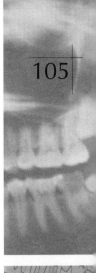

signature on file form	form that an insured completes to allow the dentist to submit an insurance claim form for a completed procedure without requiring the insured's original signature
signs and symptoms	**collectively–** the objective and subjective features of a disease that are carefully reviewed and evaluated to establish a diagnosis
	signs– characteristics that are observable by another person
	symptoms – characteristics that are described by the patient
Silastic®	material used to replace gauze, packs or other dressings
silicone	impression material that is highly accurate, dimensional stable, highly tear resistance and does not shrink or have an odor or taste
silicone spray	used as a lubricant
silver halide crystals	silver compound embedded in the emulsion on a radiograph that reacts when exposed to radiation
simultaneously	at the same time
sinus	air pocket or cavity in a bone which allows air to be warmed; helps to form sound
sinusitis	inflammation of the sinus
six-handed dentistry	dentistry performed by the operator and chairside assistant with the help from the circulating assistant
Sjögren's syndrome	chronic, inflammatory autoimmune disorder resulting in an abnormally dry mouth; the salivary glands do not produce enough saliva
slander	saying something that will harm a reputation
sloughing	refers dead tissue that is shed
slow speed handpiece	see handpiece
slurry	watery mixture of pumice, dental stone, etc.
smokeless tobacco	snuff; dip; plug; spit tobacco; chewing tobacco
socket	area of the alveolar process in which the root of a tooth is located
sodium hypochlorite	household bleach used as an intermediate-level disinfection and for rinsing during an endodontic procedure

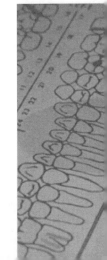

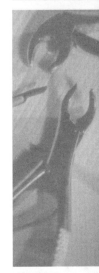

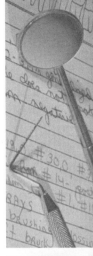

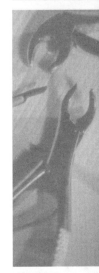

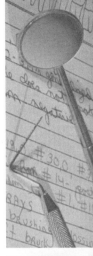

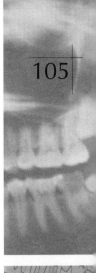

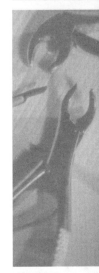

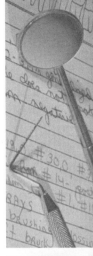

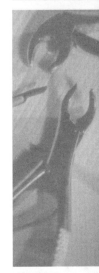

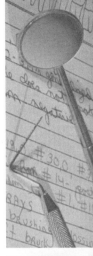

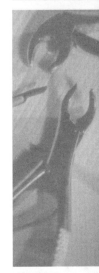

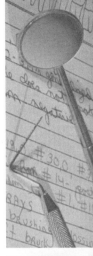

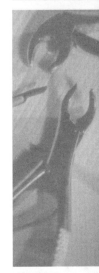

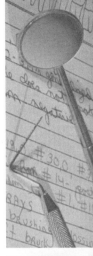

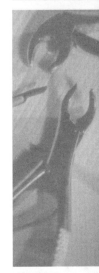

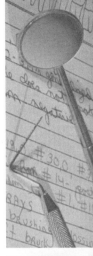

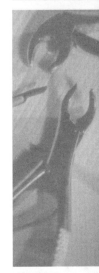

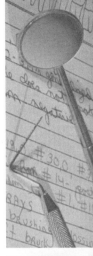

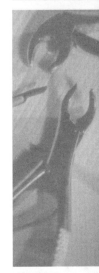

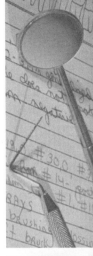

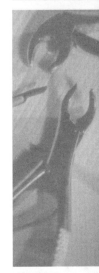

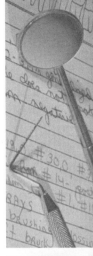

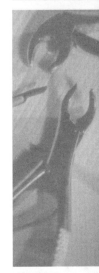

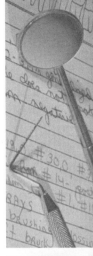

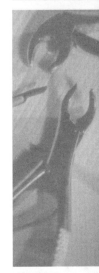

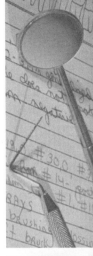

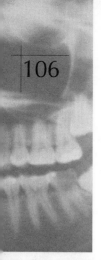
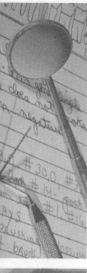
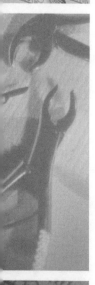
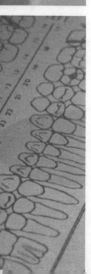

S

sodium pentathol	general anesthetic administered intravenously
sodium perborate	agent used intracoronally to bleach endodontally treated teeth
soft deposits	deposits on teeth which include food debris and plaque
soft tissue impaction	non-erupted tooth in the jaw covered by tissue only
software	programs directing to operation of a computer or specific applications
solder	to fuse by melting together with another metal of a lower melting point
solvent	liquid that can dissolve another material; i.e. dental cements
somatic	any body cells except for reproductive cells
space maintainer	wire loop soldered to a band for the maintenance of space for the future eruption of a permanent tooth
spastic contractions	sudden twitch or shrinkage of muscles involuntarily
spatter	splashing or spraying of water, prophylaxis paste, blood, saliva, etc.
spatula	flat bladed instrument used for mixing dental materials
spatulation	act of mixing material with a spatula
specimen	a sample of tissue, blood or urine, used for analysis and diagnosis; often used in reference to a biopsy
spectrum	broad range of activity
sphenoid bone	wedge-shaped bone located at the base of the skull that runs across the skull anterior to the temporal bones
sphygmomanometer	inflatable rubber bladder used to measure blood pressure
spillway	embrasure that allows food to flow from the occlusal surfaces during mastication
spirits of ammonia	mixture of ammonia, alcohol and water that is used as a stimulant for patients who have fainted (no longer recommended)
spirochete	pathogen that causes syphilis, fever and other diseases

splint	rigid appliance that fits over or is attached to teeth to broaden the area over which occlusal/incisal forces are distributed; used to support or brace teeth
spoon excavator	instrument used to remove decay and debris from teeth
spoon excavator (endodontics)	long shank instrument used to reach into root canals
spore	bacteria that has a covering which is difficult to destroy; spores are resistant to heat and require long exposure to high temperatures to kill
spore testing	the use of biological indicators (BIs) to test the use and functioning of sterilizers; see biological monitor
spot welding	see welding
spray-wipe-spray	technique used to disinfect hard surfaces
springs	bent or shaped wires that are attached to the main archwire

<u>Types</u>

coil–	spiral of wire attached to an orthodontic appliance that places pressure to expand and compress spaces
finger–	wire attached to an orthodontic appliance to tip a tooth

squamous cell carcinoma	oral lesion this is a malignant epithelial neoplasm
sputum	A mixture of saliva, mucus and other matter from the respiratory tract
stabilize	to make orderly; constant; not likely to be displaced
stain	to discolor with foreign matter; presents on the enamel surfaces of teeth

<u>Types</u>

endogenous–	develop from within tooth structure; always intrinsic; usually a discoloration of dentin reflecting through enamel
exogenous–	develop or originate from sources outside tooth; may be extrinsic; may become intrinsic
extrinsic–	occur on external surface of teeth; can be removed by polishing
intrinsic–	occur within tooth structure; cannot be removed with polishing

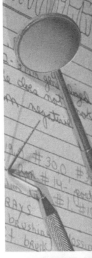

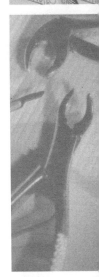

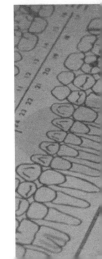

S

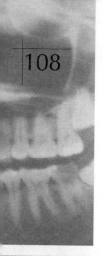
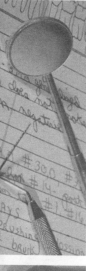
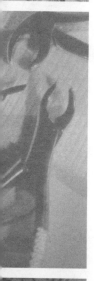
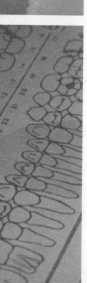

stain *(continued)*

Examples

black line stain– thin black to dark brown line of stain found just above the gingival margin

brown stain– associated with poor oral hygiene and plaque; most commonly found on the buccal surfaces of the maxillary molars and lingual surface of the mandibular incisors

chlorhexidine stain– temporary stain caused by prolonged use of chlorhexidine; is yellowish and brown in color; removed by toothbrushing and polishing

green stain– light to dark or yellowish green; is found primarily in children on the facial surface of the maxillary anterior teeth at the cervical third; contains bacteria and fungi

metallic stain– discoloration of the teeth caused by restorative materials or certain drugs

orange stain– extrinsic stain believed to be caused by bacteria related to antibiotics; found on the lingual and facial surfaces of the anterior teeth near the gingival margin

tobacco stain– brown to black stains resulting from coal tar in cigarettes and pigments from chewing tobacco; penetrates the pits and fissures in the enamel and dentin

yellow stain– associated with poor oral hygiene; most commonly found on the buccal surfaces of the maxillary molars and lingual surface of the mandibular incisors

staphylococci type of bacteria that causes what is commonly called a staph infection; potentially, the bacteria can cause a life-threatening illness should they infect a major organ; many staph infections respond to antibiotics, however, there are resistant strains emerging

staphylococcus aureus bacteria that leads to infections ranging from a severe sore throat, tonsillitis, pneumonia and endocarditis; found on skin and mucous membranes (nose and mouth) characterized by a yellow pigment

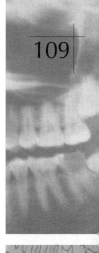

statement	bill or invoice that informs patients of the amount owed to the dentist for services rendered
static electricity	radiographic processing error that creates an image on an x-ray that looks like lightning
statute of limitations	predetermined length of time a individual has to file a complaint or law suit against another; after which time the complaint is not considered actionable
STD	acronym for sexually transmitted disease
stepwedge	device used for quality control; aluminum device that gradually increases in density to determine the penetrating ability of an x-ray
sterile	free from all forms of microorganisms
sterile water	used for irrigation in a surgical procedure
sterilize	destruction of all forms of microorganisms, including bacterial endospores
sternum	narrow, flat bone in the midline of the body on the front of the thorax
stethoscope	instrument used to hear the systolic and diastolic sounds of blood flowing while taking blood pressure
stimulus	an agent or action that causes a desired response
stippling	to have a slight bumpy or textured appearance; appearance or texture of an orange peel indicating healthy gingiva
stomatitis	inflammation of the soft tissue (gingival and lining mucosa) of the oral cavity as a result of injuries such as mechanical, chemical, thermal, bacterial, viral, electrical or radiation; reaction to allergens or a secondary manifestation of systemic disease
stone (laboratory)	gypsum material used for pouring models where more strength or accurate detail is required
stones	instrument used when maximum abrasion is needed for cutting, polishing and finishing amalgam, gold, composite and porcelain restorations
stop payment order	instruction given to a bank to stop payment on a check
strain	1) group of organisms of the same species; having the same characteristics 2) change produced within a material that occurs as the result of stress

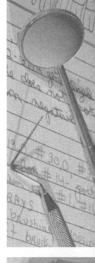
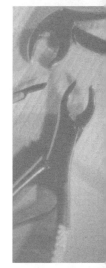
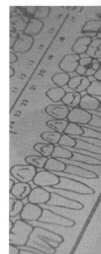

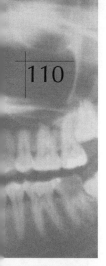
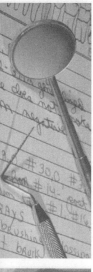
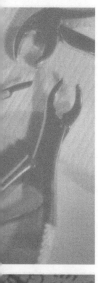
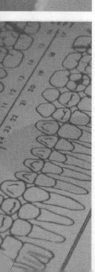

S

streptomycin	antibiotic used to fight infections
stress	a reaction within a material that can cause distortion
stripping	1) the mechanical removal of a very small amount of enamel from the mesial or distal surfaces of teeth to alleviate crowding 2) the removal of orthodontic bands at the end of treatment
study casts (models)	reproduction of a patient's dentition for the purpose of treatment planning
subacute bacterial endocarditis (SBE)	infection that may be found in patients with rheumatic or congenital heart disease
subcutaneous	beneath the surface of the skin
subgingival	below the gingival margin
Sublimaze®	see fentanyl
sublingual	under the tongue
sublingual gland	salivary gland located under the tongue that produces mucous fluid
subluxation	incomplete dislocation of a joint
submandibular gland	salivary gland located under the tongue that produces serous and mucous secretions
subperiosteal	beneath the periosteum
subpoena	legal document requiring the appearance of an individual in a court of law
subsequent	to follow close or directly after
substance abuse	compulsive use of a drug
substantivity	an attribute of some active ingredients that allows chemicals to remain on the skin after rinsing or drying, to provide an inhibitory effect on the growth of bacteria remaining on the skin
succedaneous	permanent (adult) teeth that replace primary (baby) teeth; incisors, canines and premolars, but not molars
succinylcholine	medication used to facilitate endotracheal intubation; neuromuscular blocker inducing paralysis
sulcus	space between the attached gingiva and the tooth
sulcus terminalis	shallow groove in the tongue
superbill	mutiple copy form that indicates services completed and fees

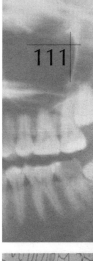

superimposed	in an x-ray, when one image is shown on top of another image
superior	upper; top
supernumerary teeth	extra teeth that can erupt or be impacted in the jaw
supernumerary tooth	extra in number; teeth are often dwarfed in shape
supervision	the active administering and overseeing of all the functioning of the dental practice and the auxiliaries employed therein; although definitions will differ from state to state, some of the most commonly used definitions for levels of supervision are:

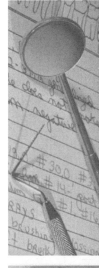

general– level of supervision that normally does not require the dentist to be physically present within the confines of the dental office, however the dentist has diagnosed the condition to be treated and has authorized the procedure

indirect– level of supervision that normally requires the dentist to be in the office, requires the dentist to prescribe a specific treatment, but does not require the dentist to see the patient either before or after treatment by the auxiliary; dentist may evaluate patient at a later time

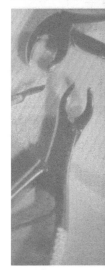

direct– level of supervision that normally requires the dentist to be in the office, requires the dentist to see the patient, prescribe treatment, and also requires the dentist to see or evaluate the patient after treatment by an auxiliary, during the same visit

personal–
1) level of supervision that requires the dentist to be in a position to observe and supervise treatment being rendered by the auxiliary
2) level of supervision requiring the dentist to be in the treatment facility, diagnose the condition to be treated, authorize the procedure, remain in the treatment facility while the procedure is being performed, and evaluate the performance before the patient is dismissed

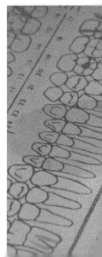

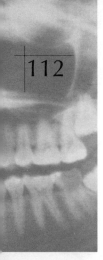

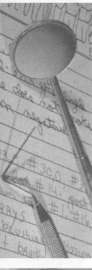

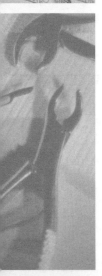

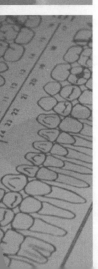

S

supine	lying on back with face up
supine position	placement of the patient in a face-up position with feet at the same level as the head
supporting structures	anatomy that supports the teeth, i.e., bone and tissue
supraeruption	eruption of a tooth beyond normal occlusion
supragingival	above the gingival margin
surface disinfectant	disinfectant that is used on hard surfaces such as countertops, operatory chairs, etc.
surgical chisel	single-beveled instrument used for removing bone; double-beveled instrument used to split teeth
surgical curette	double-ended scoop-shaped instrument used after an extraction to scrape the interior of the socket to remove diseased tissue or abscesses
surgical gowns	clothing worn by health care workers to protect against contamination from spatter and spray
surgical hand hygiene/antisepsis	handwashing or alcohol-based handscrub performed before operations by surgical personnel to reduce the number of viable microorganisms
surgical hoods	cover worn by health care workers to protect against inhalation from spatter and spray and to protect the eyes
surgical scissors	instrument used to trim soft tissue
surgical template	a guide used to shape the alveolar process and soft tissue covering to fit an immediate denture
Surgicel®	absorbent fabric that accelerates the clotting of blood
suture scissors	scissor designed with a small hook on one blade to cut only suture material
sutures	thread-like material used to close surgical incisions to promote healing and prevent bacteria and debris from entering the site; stitches

<u>Types</u>

gut–	absorbed by body; does not need to be removed
silk–	most widely used because of favorable handling characteristics and knotting security; must be removed

syncope	swooning or fainting; temporary loss of consciousness caused by inadequate blood flow to the brain; often accompanies stroke and cardiac arrhythmia

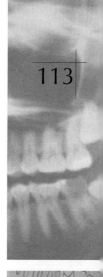

syndrome	a group of signs and symptoms that occur together and characterize a disease
synergistic	actions of two or more substances, organs or organisms that together achieve an effect of which each is individually incapable
synthetic	artificial
syphilis	sexually transmitted disease
syringe	instrument consisting of a needle, barrel and plunger used to inject fluids into the body
systemic	affecting the entire body
systemic infection	infection that affects the entire body
systemic toxicity	poisonous substance throughout person's system
systolic pressure	the first sound heard while taking blood pressure that is created when the heart forces blood through the arteries

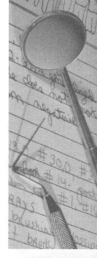

t

TB	acronym for tuberculosis
t-wave	wave in an electrocardiogram associated with ventricular activity
tachycardia	abnormally rapid heart beat; pulse rate over 100 beats per minute
tachypnea	abnormally rapid respiratory rate
tactile	sense of touch
tannic acid	an acid found in tea leaves that facilitates blood clotting
tarnish	to discolor due to exposure of air or toxins to lose luster
taste buds	cells in the tongue that allow for the sense of taste

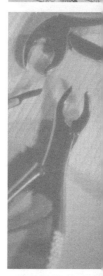

<u>Types</u>

sweet–	located at the tip
salt–	located on the anterior sides and tip
sour–	located on the sides toward the posterior
bitter–	located in the center of the dorsum toward the posterior

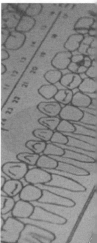

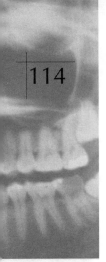
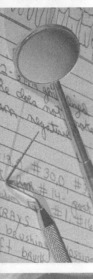
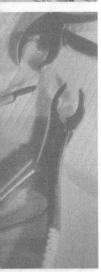
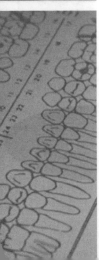

t

tax forms	forms filed with state and federal governments to indicate money earned and taxes owed

<u>Types</u>

940–	Employer's Annual federal Unemployment Tax Return–tax imposed on employers and not deducted from an employee's wage
941–	Employer's Quarterly Federal Tax Return–indicates monthly deposit for withholding taxes and social security taxes
W-2–	Wage and Tax Statement–form provided to employees indicating wages earned and all taxes removed from their annual salary
W-3–	Report of Withheld Income Tax–indicates amount of taxes withheld from employees wages
W-4–	Employee's Withholding Allowance Certificate–form completed by each employee to determine the number of deductions to be taken from their wages

tease	gently move; gently separating one item from another
temporal	near the temples of the skull
temporal bone	lateral bone of the skull located in the temporal area above each ear
temporalis muscle	muscle that elevates the mandible
temporary restoration	see provisional restoration
temporomandibular joint (TMJ)	made up of the glenoid fossa of the temporal bone, articular eminence of the temporal bone, and the condyloid process of the mandible; the left and right TMJs function in unison, move in a hinge and gliding motion and control the movements of the muscles of mastication
temporomandibular joint dysfunction (TMJD)	characterized by pain in the muscles of mastication and jaw joints, clicking and limitation in jaw movement
tensile strength	measurement of the amount of stress a material is capable of being stretched or extended before it becomes deformed
terminate	to end; to fire a staff member from employment
tetanus	infectious disease from the toxin tetanus bacillus

tetracycline	broad spectrum antibiotic
tetracycline stain	see stain
TFD	acronym for target to film distance
thermal conduction	ability of a material to conduct heat or cold
thermal sensitivity	state where tissues or teeth react with a pain sensation to hot or cold stimuli
thixotropic	the property of various gels of becoming fluid when disturbed (as by shaking)
thorax	part of the body located between the base of the neck and the diaphragm
three prong pliers	instrument used to close or adjust clasps and to bend wire
thrush	see Candidiasis
thyroid gland	gland that produces hormones that effect the metabolic rate of the body; affects physical and mental activities; required for normal growth; located at the base of the neck on the lower part of the larynx and upper part of the trachea
t.i.d.	indicates the patient is to take the prescribed medication three times a day
tinnitus	ringing, roaring, buzzing or other sounds or noises in the ears
tin oxide	very fine abrasive used to polish enamel and metallic restorations
titanium	metal used to manufacture implants, endodontic posts, orthodontic archwires, dental instruments and artificial joints
TMJ/TMD	acronym for temporomandibular joint/ dysfunction
TOD	acronym for target to film distance
tongue blade	wooden stick used to depress the tongue and view the throat
tongue thrust	movement of the tongue between the anterior teeth that can interrupt normal eruption of the teeth
tooth conditioner	see etch or acid etch

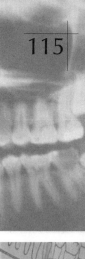

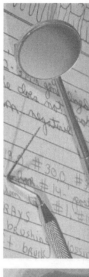

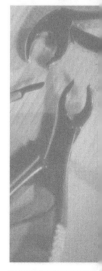

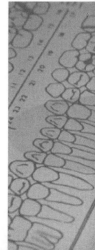

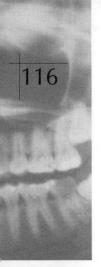

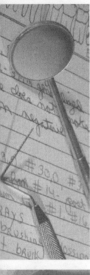

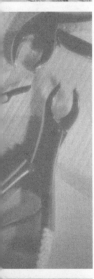

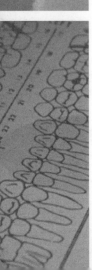

t

tooth numbering system	way of numerically and alphabetically identifying teeth

Types

International System– (or Systeme Internationale)	a two-digit code system of designating teeth for the permanent and primary dentitions; the first digit denotes the quadrant (1-4 primary, 5-8 permanent); the second digit denotes the tooth number (teeth are assigned a number from 1-8 (1-5 for primary) beginning with the central incisor
Palmer Numbering System–	number system in which the mouth is divided into quadrants (UR, UL, LL and LR) that are represented bybrackets and the teeth are assigned a number from 1–8 (1-5 for primary) beginning with the central incisor
Universal Numbering System–	numbering system where teeth are assigned a number from 1 to 32 beginning with the maxillary right third molar and ending with the mandibular right third molar

tooth positioner	device that keeps the position of the teeth after orthodontic treatment is completed (also referred to as a retainer)
topical anesthesia	gel, ointment, spray or liquid applied directly to the surface of the mucous membrane to desensitize it prior to an injection
topographical exposure	technique used to expose an occlusal radiograph
torquing	applying a twisting or turning force
torus (tori)	bulging projection of bone, usually found along the midline of the palate or on the mandibular lingual in the premolar area (either unilaterally or bilaterally); tori is the plural form of torus
toxic	harmful; poisonous
trachea	cylindrical tube that is located between the larynx and the bronchial tubes
tragus	refers to the flap of tissue on the medial of the ear opening, anterior to the external auditory canal of the ear; often used in dental radiology (along the ala of the nose) to help in positioning the head

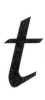

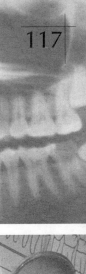

tranquilizer	a drug that calms without affecting consciousness
transfuse	inject blood from one person to another
translucent	ability to transmit light but diffuse an image
transmission	to send from one person, place or thing to another; to cause to spread, to pass on

Types

airborne transmission (droplet)–	mode of infection caused by droplets of moisture which may contain bacteria or viruses
bloodborne transmission–	mode of infection caused by direct or indirect contact with blood; transmission of pathogens through the blood and body fluids
direct contact transmission–	contact with a lesion, organism or debris (indirect contact) or contamination through instruments, equipment or supplies, (inhalation) or aerosolization from blood or saliva
indirect contact transmission–	contamination through handling contaminated instruments or touching contaminated surfaces
parenteral transmission–	contamination through the skin and is commonly associated with injections

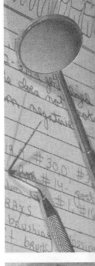

traumatize	to injure physically or mentally
treatment plan	plan developed by the dentist for a patient which includes diagnosis and recommended course of treatment
treatment record	record for each patient which indicates all dental treatment rendered and recommendations provided to a patient
Trendelenberg postion	placement of a patient in a position on his/her back where his/her head is lower than her/his feet with the legs elevated
triclosan	a chemical, chlorophenol, used in oral rinses to stop or limit odor and in antiseptic soap to reduce the number of organisms
trifurcated	three roots
trismus	spasms of the muscles of mastication creating an inability to open the mouth

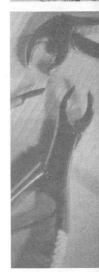

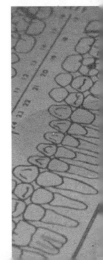

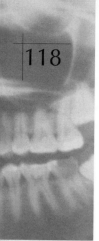
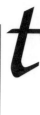
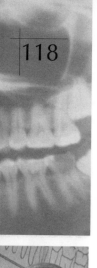
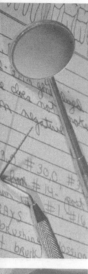
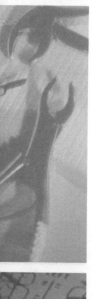

t

trituration	the act of mixing using pressure; see amalgamation
tubehead	part of the x-ray machine that houses the two main components of the x-ray machine, the cathode and anode
tuberculocidal	agent that has the ability to kill the tuberculosis virus
tuberculosis (TB)	disease that most often settles in the lungs which is spread by airborne particles from coughing, sneezing, salivary contact, and cross contamination
tuberculosis skin test	test performed to determine if an individual may have been in contact with or infected by the tuberculosis bacterium
tuberosity	elevation from the surface; protrusion of a bone
tumor	see neoplasm
Tweed-loop pliers	instrument that forms loops and springs in orthodontic wire
Tx	acronym for treatment

u

UCR	see usual, customary and reasonable fee
ulcer	an inflammation on the skin or on a mucous surface of the body; causes gradual disintegration of the tissue
ulceration	result of an ulcer
ulcerative	ability to become affected with an ulcer
ultrasonic cleaner	machine that transmits high energy and high frequency vibrations to a chemical solution used to remove debris from instruments and removable appliances
unconscious	lack of sensory perception which results in a lack of subjective experiences
underexposure	film that appears light because of improper exposure settings or from a position indicating device (PID) that was not positioned close enough to the patient
unit dosing	quantity sufficient for one dose; packaging materials in single-use portions
universal forceps	instrument used to remove teeth from the left or right side of the same arch

universal precautions	methods employed to maintain an aseptic field and to prevent cross contamination; treating each patient as potentially infectious
unsaturated chemical vapor sterilizer	sterilizer that uses a combination of chemicals to create a vapor for sterilizing
urinalysis	microscopic examination of urine to determine if an abnormal state exists within the body
urticaria	rash; hives
user	one who uses
usual, customary and reasonable fee (UCR)	fee that is determined by an insurance carrier from information gathered from dentists in a geographical region; insurance reimbursements are based on UCRs
utility gloves	see nitrile gloves

VA	acronym for vertical angle
vaccination	inoculation with a vaccine to protect against disease
vaccine	agent prepared to produce an active immunity that usually kills microbes or strains of microbes that induce antibody production without producing disease
vacuum mixer	equipment that mixes gypsum using suction, leaving the mix free of air bubbles
Valium®	see diazepam
vapors	vaporized substance that emits an odor; gaseous state of any substance; visable discharge of fine particles of a liquid
varix	an enlarged tortuous (twisted) vein, artery, or lymph vessel such as a varicose vein; a condition primarily in the elderly
vasoconstrictor	substance that constricts blood vessels around an injection site creating a reduction of blood flow
vasodilator	drug that increases the diameter of blood vessels
vein	blood vessel through which blood flows toward the heart
veneer	covering for the facial surface of teeth that is fabricated from procelain, gold or acrylic or composite resin

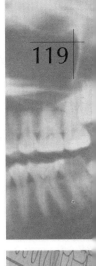
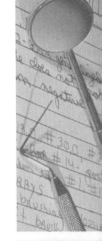
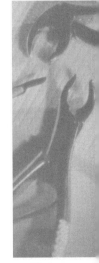
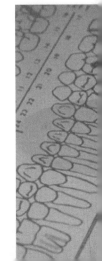

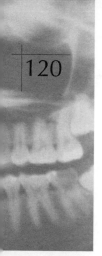

v

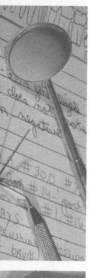

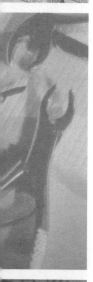

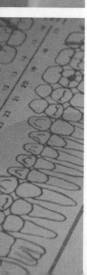

ventral	toward the abdomen; bottom surface such as the under surface of the tongue
verification	to affirm validity; to demonstrate something is true or accurate
ventilate	to circulate with new air and to expel contaminated air
Versed®	see midazolam
versus	against; in comparison to
vertical	in an up and down direction
vertical angulation	placement of the central beam in an up or down position
vertical dimension	space provided by the teeth in normal occlusion; a measurement of the face at the midline
vessel	a tube, duct or canal that carries fluids of the body
vestibule	pocket located between the teeth and gingiva and the lips and cheeks
vestibuloplasty	restoration of the alveolar ridge height by lowering the muscles attached to the buccal, lingual and labial aspects of the jaw
vial	small container for medicines or chemicals
virulent	extremely harmful; very infectious
virus	infectious agent that lives within a host cell, that transforms the cell and releases it into the body to infect other cells
viscosity	degree of ability to flow; thickness of a liquid
viscous	thick liquid
visibly soiled hands	hands showing visible dirt or visibly contaminated with proteinaceous body substances; i.e., blood, fecal material or urine
vital signs	signs of life; including temperature, blood pressure, respiration and pulse rate
vitality	level of life
vitalometer	instrument that provides a current to create an electrical stimulus to measure vitality in a tooth
vitamin A	vitamin that is essential for normal growth and development
vitamin B	vitamin that effects growth appetite, gastrointestinal, nervous and endocrine systems; is necessary for carbohydrate metabolism

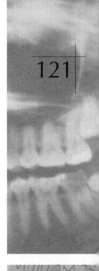

vitamin B1	vitamin that provides thiamine; essential for normal metabolism of carbohydrates and fats
vitamin B2	vitamin that provides riboflavin; essential for tissue repair
vitamin C	vitamin recommended for the prevention and treatment of colds
vitamin D	vitamin that is essential for calcium and phosphorus metabolism
vitamin K	vitamin that helps to eliminate prolonged bleeding
vomitus	material ejected by the body when vomiting; the product of regurgitation; see regurgitate

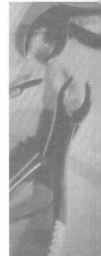

warfarin sodium	oral anticoagulant; indirectly stops or slows clotting of blood; trade names include Coumadin®, Panwarfin® and Sofarin®
washing	step in radiographic processing that removes any remaining chemicals
wasting	loss of strength or size
water/powder ratio	amount of water needed in relationship to a given amount of powder in order to reach a desired consistency
waterline contamination	presence of biofilm on the inner surface of water lines
Waters view	radiographic exposure used to view the maxillary sinuses
wavelength	distance between the peaks of waves in x-rays

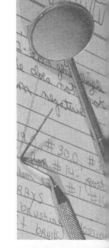

Types

long–	low energy and frequency wavelengths that are unsuitable for exposing radiographs
short–	high energy and high frequency wavelengths with high penetrating power; known as hard radiation used to expose radiographs

wbc	acronym for white blood cells
wear facets	flat spots ground into the occlusal surfaces and incisal edges of teeth from chewing and grinding
wedge	device used to seal the gingival margin of a cavity preparation to prevent overhangs and to maintain proximal contact

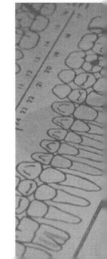

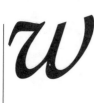

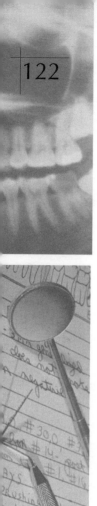

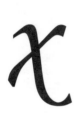

W

Weingart utility plier	instrument used for placing archwires
welding (spot)	process used to attach brackets onto orthodontic bands
wicking	absorption of a liquid by capillary action along a thread or through the material; i.e. penetration of liquid through undetected holes in a glove
wnl	acronym for within normal limits
work practice controls	the Occupational Safety and Health Administration (OSHA) identifies these as techniques or practices that reduce the possibility of exposure to pathogenic organisms by changing the manner in which a task is performed; i.e., a one-handed scoop technique for recapping a needle

X

X-radiation	the energy produced within the tubehead of an x-ray unit; another term for x-rays
x-ray control panel	panel that contains the controls for turning the radiographic equipment on and off and for adjusting the kVp and mA
Xylocaine®	see lidocaine

Z

zinc oxide eugenol (ZOE)	a material used for the sedative effect on the pulp; type I is used for cementing temporary restorations; type II can be used for cementing permanent restorations; see intermediate restorative material
zinc phosphate cement	permanent cement; thermal insulating cement base
zirconium silicate	abrasive used for removal of stain and for polishing gold restorations, exposed dentin, composites and enamel
ZOE	acronym for zinc oxide-eugenol

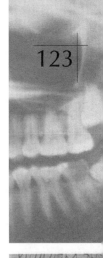

zone of activity   in four-handed dentistry, the areas of work (for right handed operators) as they relate to the face of a clock.

12:00–2:00 **Static Zone–**	area of least activity where infrequently used instruments and equipment are located
2:00–4:00 **(sometimes 5:00)** **Assistant's Zone–**	area dominated by the assistant and where frequently used instruments and supplies are located
4:00 (5:00)–8:00 **Transfer Zone**	area where instruments and materials are transferred to the operator
8:00–12:00 **Operator's Zone–**	area that allows the operator to move freely in order to achieve the most complete access and visibility for the operator

zygoma   forms the cheek bones; also known as the malar bone

zygomatic arch   bowlike prominence created at the side of the head by the temporal process of the zygoma uniting with the zygomatic process of the temporal bone; also known as the cheek

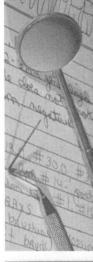

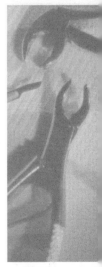

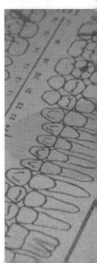

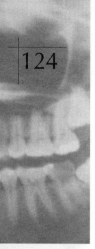

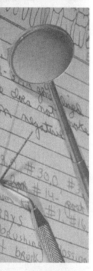

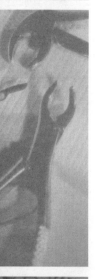

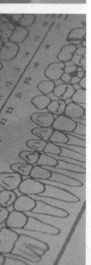

APPENDIX A

Reprinted with permission of the Joint Commission on Accreditation of Healthcare Organizations and the American Dental Association

Academy for Implants and Transplants (AIT)
Founded: 1972. Headquarters: Springfield, VA. Purpose: To encourage and promote the art and science of implant and transplant dentistry. It serves dentists who assist generalist dentists in the field of implants and transplants.

Academy for Sports Dentistry (ASD)
Founded 1983. Headquarters: Iowa City, IA. Purpose: To foster research, development, and education in all sciences related to sports dentistry and its relationship to the body as a whole. Membership comprises dentists physicians and athletic trainers.

Academy of Dentistry for the Handicapped (ADH)
Founded: 1952. Headquarters: Chicago, IL. Purpose: To promote dental education research and legislation to improve the health and sensitivity of parents, advocates, and related professional groups. Members include dentists, dental hygienists, dental assistants, and allied health professionals specializing in improving the oral health of persons with special dental needs.

Academy of General Dentistry (AGD)
Founded: 1952. Headquarters: Chicago, IL. Purpose: To serve the needs and to represent the interests of general dentists and to foster their continued proficiency through quality continuing dental education in order to better serve the public.

Academy of Operative Dentistry (AOD)
Founded 1972. Headquarters: Menomonie, WI. Purpose: To ensure quality education in operative dentistry. Members include dentists and persons in allied industries interested in quality education in operative dentistry.

American Academy of Dental Group Practice (AADGP)
Founded: 1973. Headquarters: Palatine, IL. Purpose: To improve level of service provided by members through exchange and expansion of ideas and techniques for patient treatment. It serves dentists and dental group practices interested in practice management and treatment in group practice settings.

American Academy of Dental Practice Administration (AADPA)
Founded: 1958. Headquarters: Palatine, IL. Purpose: To promote the efficient administration of dental practice.

American Academy of Oral and Maxillofacial Pathology (AAOMP)
Founded: 1946. Headquarters: Naperville, IL. Purpose: To serve oral pathologists who study and treat diseases of the mouth and oral cavity. Formerly: American Academy of Oral Pathology (1994).

American Academy of Oral and Maxillofacial Radiology (AAOMR)
Founded: 1949. Headquarters: Jackson, MS. Purpose: To promote and advance the art and science of oral and maxillofacial radiology, to provide the opportunity for professionals in oral and maxillofacial radiology to communicate and achieve recognition of their work, and to seek mutual understanding and appreciation of radiology among the medical and dental professions.

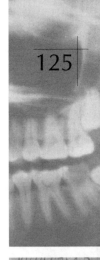

American Academy of Oral Medicine (AAOM)
Founded: 1946. Headquarters: Arlington, VA. Purpose: To promote the study of the cause, prevention, and control of diseases of the teeth and to foster better scientific understanding between the fields of dentistry and medicine. Members include dental educators, specialists, general dentists, and physicians interested in the study of diseases of the mouth.

American Academy of Pediatric Dentistry (AAPD)
Founded: 1947. Headquarters: Chicago, IL. Purpose: To advance pediatric dentistry through practice, education, and research. It serves teachers and researchers in pediatric dentistry and dentists whose practice is limited to children.

American Academy of Periodontology (AAP)
Founded: 1914. Headquarters: Chicago, IL. Purpose: To advance the art and science of periodontics, improve the periodontal health of the public, and serve the interests of the members of the academy. Membership mainly consists of dental professionals, the majority of whom are periodontists-a dental specialist who is an expert in the prevention, diagnosis, and treatment of diseases affecting the gums and supporting structures of the teeth and in the placement and maintenance of dental implants.

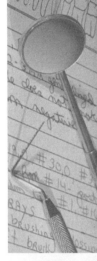

American Academy of Restorative Dentistry (AARD)
Founded: 1928. Headquarters: Colorado Springs, CO. Purpose: To research application of the treatment of the natural teeth to restore and maintain a healthy functioning mouth as part of a healthy body. It serves dentists practicing restorative dentistry and educators.

American Association for Dental Research (AADR)
Founded: 1972. Headquarters: Washington, DC. Purpose: To promote better dental health and research activities. It is composed of dentists, researchers, dental schools, and dental products-manufacturing companies.

American Association of Dental Consultants (AADC)
Founded: 1977. Headquarters: Lawrence, KS. Purpose: To operate a certification program. It serves dental insurance consultants and others interested in dental insurance plans from administrative and design perspectives.

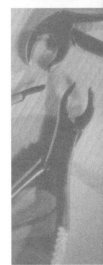

American Association of Dental Examiners (AADE)
Founded: 1883. Headquarters: Chicago, IL. Purpose: To assist member agencies with problems relating to state dental board examinations and licensure, and enforcement of the state dental practice act. It serves present and past members of state dental examining boards and board administrators.

American Association of Endodontists (AAE)
Founded: 1943. Headquarters: Chicago, IL. Purpose: Promotes the exchange of ideas on the scope of the specialty of endodontics; stimulates endodontic research studies among its members; and encourages the highest standard of care in the practice of endodontics. It serves dentists engaged in clinical practice, teaching, and research in endodontics.

American Association of Entrepreneurial Dentists (AAED)
Founded: 1983. Headquarters: Tupelo, MS. Purpose: To inform the public, dentists, educators, and manufacturing companies of new and beneficial techniques, products, and services; coordinates the review of specifications for dental materials and products by regulatory agencies; evaluates and represents new ideas and products to manufacturing companies at convention trade expositions; and provides lists of foreign dental dealers and buyers. It is composed of dentists and other dental professionals involved in research, industry, manufacturing, marketing, publication, and other entrepreneurial activities.

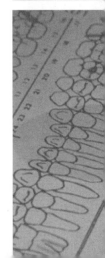

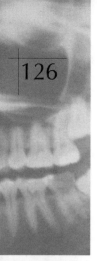
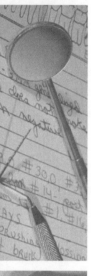
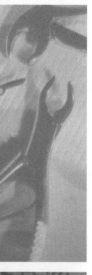
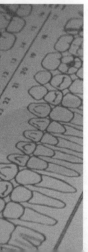

American Association of Functional Orthodontics (AAFO)
Founded: 1982. Headquarters: Winchester, VA. Purpose: To serve its membership by being a source of the latest and best information available anywhere on the subject of functional appliance therapy and temporomandibular joint therapy through exclusive original articles published in its journal. It serves orthodontists, pediatric dentists and general practitioners from throughout the United States, Canada, and over 20 other foreign countries.

American Association of Hospital Dentists (AAHD)
Founded: 1927. Headquarters: Chicago, IL. Purpose: To promote dental education programs in hospitals.

American Association of Oral and Maxillofacial Surgeons (AAOMS)
Founded: 1918. Headquarters: Rosemont, IL. Purpose: To promote the highest quality of patient care and education, to maintain high professional standards of practice through continuing education, and to foster and support specialty research. It serves dentists specializing in disease diagnosis and surgical and adjunctive treatment of diseases, injuries, and defects of the oral and maxillofacial region.

American Association of Orthodontists (AAO)
Founded: 1901. Headquarters: St. Louis, MO. Purpose: To advance the art and science of orthodontics through continuing education, encouragement of research, provision of information to the public, and cooperation with other health groups. Members include orthodontists.

American Association of Public Health Dentistry (AAPHD)
Founded: 1937. Headquarters: Richmond, VA. Purpose: To improve total health for all citizens through the development and support of effective programs of oral health promotion and disease prevention through the promotion of effective efforts in disease prevention, health promotion and service delivery; education of the public, health professionals and decision makers regarding the importance of oral health to total well-being; and expansion of the knowledge base of dental public health and fostering competency in its practice. AAPHD membership is open to all individuals concerned with improving the oral health of the public.

American Association of Stomatologists (AAS)
Founded: 1985. Headquarters: Freehold, NJ. Purpose: To establish oral diagnosis, radiology, and medicine as recognized specialties in dentistry. It serves coordinating organizations representing the American Academy of Oral Medicine and the Organization of Teachers of Oral Diagnosis.

American Association of Women Dentists (AAWD)
Founded: 1921. Headquarters: Chicago, IL. Purpose: To encourage women to pursue an academic degree in dentistry and to advance the status of women in the dental profession. It serves women dentists and dental students.

American Board of Dental Public Health (ABDPH)
Founded: 1950. Headquarters: Gainesville, FL. Purpose: To investigate the qualifications of, administer examinations to, and certify as diplomates dentists specializing in dental public health. Sponsored by the American Association of Public Health.

American Board of Endodontics (ABE)
Founded: 1964. Headquarters: Chicago, IL. Purpose: Certifies dentists who have successfully completed study and training in an advanced endodontics education program accredited by the Commission on Dental Accreditation of the American Dental Association and who have successfully completed the examinations administered by the board.

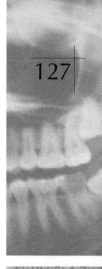

American Board of Oral and Maxillofacial Surgery (ABOMS)
Founded: 1946. Headquarters: Chicago, IL. Purpose: Certifies as diplomates dentists specializing in oral and maxillofacial surgery.

American Board of Oral Pathology (ABOP)
Founded: 1948. Headquarters: Tampa, FL. Purpose: To arrange, conduct, and control examinations to determine the competence of applicants wishing to be certified in oral pathology.

American Board of Orthodontics (ABO)
Founded: 1929. Headquarters: St. Louis, MO. Purpose: Investigates the qualifications of, administers examinations to, and certifies as diplomates dentists specializing in orthodontics.

American Board of Pediatric Dentistry (ABPD)
Founded: 1940. Headquarters: Carmel, IN. Purpose: Investigates the qualifications of, administers examinations to, and certifies as diplomates dentists specializing in the care of children.

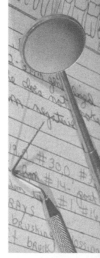

American Board of Periodontology (ABP)
Founded: 1939. Headquarters: Baltimore, MD. Purpose: Conducts examinations to determine the qualifications and competence of dentists who voluntarily apply for certification as diplomates in the field of periodontology (periodontics).

American College of Dentists (ACD)
Founded: 1920. Headquarters: Gaithersburg, MD. Purpose: To conduct educational and research programs. Members include dentists and other individuals interested in advancing the standards of the profession of dentistry.

American College of Oral and Maxillofacial Surgeons (ACOMS)
Founded: 1975. Headquarters: San Antonio, TX. Purpose: To enhance the level of patient care through the furthering of research and education in OMS surgery and to preserve and promote the integrity of the specialty and its advancement. The ACOMS sponsors educational programs, research activities, and fellowships as a service both to members and to the profession at large. As a multidisciplinary group, it stresses seeking input from other disciplines.

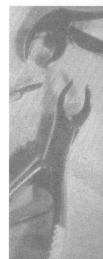

American College of Prosthodontists (ACP)
Founded: 1970. Headquarters: Chicago, IL. Purpose: to encourage educational activities. It serves dentists specializing in prosthetics who are either board certified, board prepared, or under training in an approved graduate or residency program.

American Dental Assistants Association (ADAA)
Founded: 1923. Headquarters: Chicago, IL. Purpose: National membership organization for dental assistants. Sponsors workshops and seminars for individuals employed as dental assistants in dental offices, clinics, hospitals, or institutions; instructors of dental assistants; and dental students.

American Dental Association (ADA)
Founded: 1859. Headquarters: Chicago, IL. Purpose: To promote the public's health through commitment of member dentists to provide quality oral health care accessible to everyone and to promote the profession of dentistry by enhancing the integrity and ethics of the profession, strengthening the patient-dentist relationship, and making membership the foundation of successful practice. The ADA fulfills its public and professional mission by providing services and through its initiatives in education, research, advocacy, and the development of standards. ADA programs and products include the Survey Center (SC), which monitors trends; the ADA Seal of Acceptance, which indicates a dental product's safety and effectiveness; and a direct reimbursement dental benefits plan kit. The ADA is a member organization of the Joint Commission.

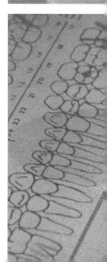

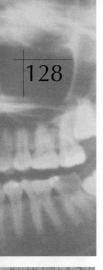

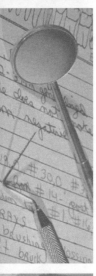

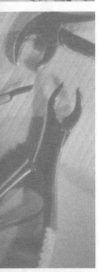

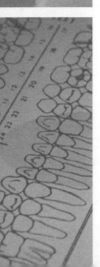

American Dental Education Association (ADEA)
(formerly the American Association of Dental Schools (AADS)
Founded: 1923. Headquarters: Washington, DC. Purpose: To lead the dental education community in addressing the contemporary issues influencing education, research, and the health of the public. Its members include all U.S. and Canadian dental schools, advanced dental education programs, hospital dental education programs, allied dental education programs, corporations, faculty, and students.

American Dental Hygienists' Association (ADHA)
Founded: 1923. Headquarters: Chicago, IL. Purpose: To maintain an accrediting service through the American Dental Association's Commission on Dental Accreditation. It serves licensed dental hygienists possessing a degree or certificate in dental hygiene granted by an accredited school of dental hygiene.

American Dental Society of Anesthesiology (ADSA)
Founded: 1953. Headquarters: Chicago, IL. Purpose: To encourage study and progress in dental anesthesiology. It serves dentists and physicians.

American Dental Trade Association (ADTA)
Founded: 1882. Headquarters: Alexandria, VA. Purpose: To conduct sales and training programs. It serves dental laboratories and manufacturers and distributors of dental instruments, supplies, and equipment.

American Endodontic Society (AES)
Founded: 1969. Headquarters: Fullerton, CA. Purpose: To promote and provide educational and scientific information on simplified root canal therapy for the generalist dentist. It serves dentists.

American Educational Research Association (AERA)
Founded: 1916. Headquarters: Washington, DC. Purpose: To improve the educational process by encouraging scholarly inquiry related to education and by promoting the documentation and practical application of research results.

American Equilibration Society (AES)
Founded: 1955. Headquarters: Morton Grove, IL. Purpose: Increase study and proficiency in the diagnosis and treatment of occlusive and temporomandibular joint disorders. It serves 1,500 dentists, orthodontists, oral surgeons, and physicians.

American Heart Association (AHA)
Founded: 1924. Headquarters: Dallas, TX. Purpose: To reduce premature death and disability from cardiovascular diseases and stroke through support of research, education, and community service programs serving physicians, scientists, and laypersons. The AHA, also sometimes called the Heart Fund, is a community-based organization with state and metropolitan affiliates. It is financed entirely by voluntary contributions from the public, principally during the Heart Campaign held each year in February. Professional and scientific activities include development of clinical practice guidelines and provision of training systems to teach emergency care procedures.

American National Standards Institute (ANSI)
Founded: 1918. Headquarters: New York, NY. Purpose: To provide a clearinghouse for nationally coordinated voluntary standards for fields ranging from information technology to building construction; to give status as American National standards to standards developed by agreement from all groups interested in various areas; and to provide information on foreign standards and represent U.S. interests in international standardization work. It serves industrial firms, trade associations, technical societies, labor organizations, consumer organizations, and government agencies.

American Orthodontic Society (AOS)
Founded: 1974. Headquarters: Dallas, TX. Purpose: To render orthodontic information readily available to ethical dentists and monitoring third-party services and government programs and to offer courses in orthodontic techniques. It serves general and pediatric dentists.

American Prosthodontic Society (APS)
Founded: 1928. Headquarters: Chicago, IL. Purpose: A professional society of dentists interested in prosthodontics.

American Red Cross National Headquarters (ARC)
Founded: 1881. Headquarters: Washington, DC. Purpose: To provide care for the wounded, sick, and homeless in wartime, according to the terms of the Geneva Convention of 1864, and now also during and following natural disasters; to conduct research programs; and to maintain local chapters that provide speakers. The emblem of the organization is a Geneva cross or a red Greek cross on a white background.

American Society for Geriatric Dentistry (ASGD)
Founded: 1965. Headquarters: Chicago, IL. Purpose: To promote continuing education of the practitioner of geriatric dentistry; nursing home administrators and personnel; and dental hygienists, nurses, and students. It serves dentists, dental hygienists, and dental students interested in oral health care for older adults in all health care settings (acute care, ambulatory care, home care, and long term care).

Association for Professionals in Infection Control (APIC)
Founded: 1972. Headquarters: Washington, DC. Purpose: To promote quality research and standardization of practices and procedures; to develop communications among members; and to assess and influence legislation related to the field. Members include physicians, nurses, epidemiologists, microbiologists, medical technicians, pharmacists, and sanitarians interested in infection control. Formerly: Association for Practitioners in Infection Control and Epidemiology (1994).

American Society of Dentistry for Children (ASDC)
Founded: 1927. Headquarters: Chicago, IL. Purpose: To conduct specialized education and research programs and provide placement service for graduates in dentistry. It serves general practitioners and specialists interested in dentistry for children.

American Society of Forensic Odontology (ASFO)
Founded: 1966. Headquarters: Chicago, IL. Purpose: To conduct research and specialized education programs. It serves individuals interested in the field of forensic dentistry.

American Society of Maxillofacial Surgeons (ASMS)
Founded: 1947. Headquarters: Arlington Heights, IL. Purpose: To stimulate and advance knowledge of the science and art of maxillofacial surgery and improve and elevate the standard of practice. Members include physicians and dentists who have at least five years of recognized graduate training and experience in maxillofacial surgery.

Association of Schools of Allied Health Professions (ASAHP)
Founded: 1967. Headquarters: Washington, DC. Purpose: To enhance the effectiveness of education for the allied health professions. Provides a forum which links leaders in allied health education with state and national policy makers in government, business, and industry in efforts to effect relevant and appropriate changes in health care policy. Members include administrators, educators, and others who are concerned with critical issues affecting allied health education.

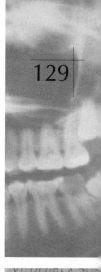
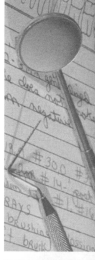
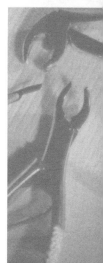
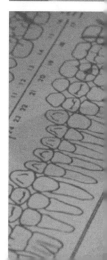

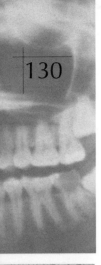
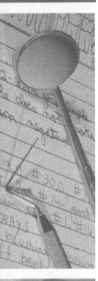

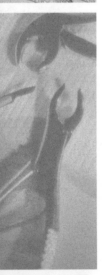

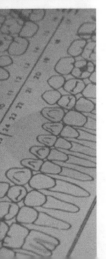

Association of State and Territorial Dental Directors (ASTDD)

Founded: unknown. Headquarters: Minneapolis, MN. Purpose: To provide a forum for consideration of dental health administrative problems for directors of state and territorial dental programs.

Bureau of Health Professions

Provides national leadership in coordinating, evaluating, and supporting the development of the nation's health personnel. It promotes quality assurance activities, operates the National Practitioner Data Bank and the Vaccine Injury Compensation Program, funds educational services and training for health professions faculty, promotes equity in access to health services and health careers for the disadvantaged, and funds regional centers to train health professionals and faculty in the counseling, diagnosis, and management of HIV/AIDS-infected individuals.

Centers for Disease Control and Prevention (CDC)

Founded: 1973. Headquarters: Atlanta, GA. Purpose: To protect the public health of the nation by providing leadership and direction in the prevention and control of diseases and other preventable conditions and responding to public health emergencies. It administers national programs for the prevention and control of communicable and vector-borne diseases, injury, and other preventable conditions; directs and enforces foreign quarantine activities and regulations; provides consultation and assistance in upgrading the performance of public health and clinical laboratories; and organizes and implements a National Health Promotion Program. It administers the National Nosocomial Infections Surveillance (NNIS) system, the only source of national surveillance data on nosocomial infections in the United States. A new collaborative initiative begun with Glaxo Wellcome, Inc, and Merck & Co. Inc, is the HIV Postexposure Prophylaxis (PEP) Registry. The CDC is composed of 11 major operating components: Epidemiology Program Office (EPO); International Health Program Office (IHPO); National Center for Chronic Disease Prevention and Health Promotion (NCCDPHP); National Center for Environmental Health (NCEH); National Center for Health Statistics (NCHS); National Center for HIV, ST [sexually transmitted disease], and TB [tuberculosis] Prevention (NCHSTP); National Center for Infectious Diseases (NCID), which includes the Hospital Infections Program (HIP); National Center for Injury Prevention and Control (NCIPC); National Center for Prevention Services; National Immunization Program (NIP) Office, which includes the Advisory Committee on Immunization Practices (ACIP); National Institute for Occupational Safety and Health (NIOSH); and Public Health Practice Program (PHPP) Office

College of Diplomates of the American Board of Orthodontics (CDABO)

Founded: Atlanta, GA by John K. Ottley, Jr. Headquarters: San Francisco, CA. Purpose: Promotes self-evaluation and ongoing professional improvement among orthodontists and conducts seminars. Members are diplomats of the American Board of Orthodontics who qualify by passing extra examinations.

Commission on Dental Accreditation

Founded: The Commission on Dental Accreditation, the successor of the Council on Dental Education which had conducted the accreditation program since 1937, began operating in 1975. Headquarters: American Dental Association Headquarters, Chicago, IL. Purpose: The Commission on Dental Accreditation is concerned with the educational quality of dental, allied dental and advanced and specialty dental education programs in the United States. Through its accreditation activities, the Commission attempts to foster educational excellence, supports programmatic self-improvement and assures the general public of the ongoing availability of quality dental care. The Commission received its accreditation authority from the acceptance of the dental community and by being recognized by the United State Department of Education (USDE). The Commission serves as the only nationally-recognized accrediting body for dentistry and related dental fields, and accredits more than 1,300 programs in the disciplines within its purview.

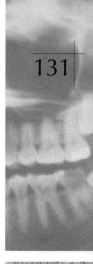

Council on Dental Education and Licensure (CDEL)
Founded: 1937. Headquarters: Chicago, IL The Council on Dental Education and Licensure (CDEL) is the ADA agency dedicated to promoting high quality and effective processes of dental education, dental licensure and credentialing in the United States. The CDEL, through its tripartite representative structure (ADA, ADEA, AADE), fulfills its mission by:
1) monitoring and disseminating information on dental education and licensure issues,
2) conducting studies and providing recommendations to the ADA's policy-making bodies on these matters,
3) serving as liaison to related organizations which also serve dental education and licensure, and
4) implementing the directions of the Board of Trustees and the House of Delegates of the ADA.

Delta Dental Plans Association (DDPA)
Founded: 1954. Headquarters: Oak Brook, IL. Purpose: Carries dental, oral healthcare, and medical benefits for U.S. citizens. A new educational program, PANDA (Prevent Abuse and Neglect through Dental Awareness), teaches dental health professionals how to recognize child abuse. Members are made up of local, nonprofit Delta Dental Plans that provide groups with dental benefits coverage.

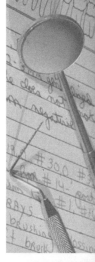

Dental Assisting National Board, Inc. (DANB)
Founded: 1948. Headquarters: Chicago, IL. Purpose: To promote the public good by providing credentialingservices to the dental community. DANB measures the success of this mission by providing: properly governed, financially secure and administratively sound organization; valid dental assisting credentialing examinations; dental assisting recertification process integrity; visible, valuable, accessible DANB credentials; other testing services for groups within the dental community, as deemed appropriate and information services for the oral healthcare community related to dental assisting credentialing and recertification. DANB is an independent national testing organization recognized by the American Dental Association and other national and state agencies for the administration of national certification examinations and state-specific examinations for dental assistants. The national certifications available are the Certified Dental Assistant, Certified Orthodontic Assistant, Certified Dental Practice Management Administrator. Although the Certified Oral and Maxillofacial Surgery Assistant examination is no longer offered, the credential continues to be recognized.

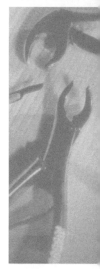

Department of Veterans Affairs (VA)
Founded: 1930. Headquarters: Washington, DC. Purpose: To operate programs to benefit veterans and members of their families, including disability and death benefits, pensions, education, rehabilitation, and a medical care program incorporating nursing homes, clinics, and medical centers. The VA comprises three organizations that administer veterans programs; the Veterans Health Administration (VHA), the Veterans Benefits Administration (VBA), and the National Cemetery system. Each organization has a central office and field facilities. The VHA conducts both individual medical and health care delivery research projects and multihospital research programs in its VA Medical Centers (VAMCs), and it assists in the education and training of physicians and many other health care professionals. The VHA operates the Civilian Health and Medical Program (CHAMPVA), which provides dependents of certain veterans with medical care supplied by non-VA institutions and physicians. The VBA operates the Vocational Rehabilitation Service for disable veterans and their immediate families and to certain handicapped dependents.

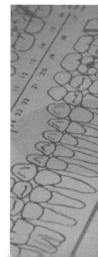

Drug Enforcement Administration (DEA)
Founded: 1973. Headquarters: Arlington, VA. Purpose: To serve as the lead federal agency in enforcing narcotics and controlled substances laws and regulations. It enforces the provisions of the controlled substances and chemical diversion and trafficking laws and regulations of the United States.

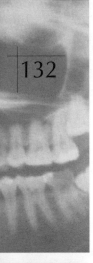
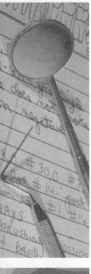
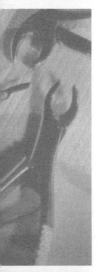
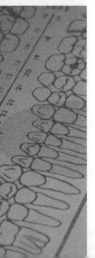

Environmental Protection Agency (EPA)
Founded: 1970. Headquarters: Washington, DC. Purpose: To protect and enhance the environment currently and for future generations to the fullest extent possible under the laws enacted by Congress and through cooperation with state and local governments. The EPA works to control and abate pollution in the air, water, solid waste, pesticides, radiation, and toxic substances.

Federal Communications Commission (FCC)
Founded: 1934. Headquarters: Washington, DC. Purpose: An independent U.S. government agency, directly responsible to Congress, charged with regulatory interstate and international communications by radio, television, wire, satellite, and cable.

Federation of Prosthodontic Organizations (FPO)
Founded: 1965. Headquarters: Chicago, IL. Purpose: To improve prosthodontic service rendered to the public and to improve communication among members and other organizations. Members are organizations of dentists.

Federation of Special Care Organizations and Dentistry
Founded: 1965. Headquarters: Chicago, IL. Purpose: To improve the effectiveness of health care providers in providing quality patient care, especially for patients who for reasons of medical diagnosis, disabilities, or frailties prevalent in advanced age require special care and/or special settings for dental care. The group is affiliated with the Academy of Dentistry for Persons with Disabilities, American Association of Hospital Dentists, and American Society for Geriatric Dentistry.

Food and Drug Administration (FDA)
Founded: 1931. Headquarters: Washington, DC. Purpose: To protect the health of the nation against impure and unsafe foods, drugs, and cosmetics, and other potential hazards. It develops and administers programs concerning safety, effectiveness, and labeling of all drug, food, and cosmetic products and all medical devices for human use, and it operates MedWatch, the FDA Medical Products Reporting Program (supported by more than 120 organizations called MedWatch, Partners). In February 1997, the FDA issued rules prohibiting sale and promotion of cigarettes, loose cigarette tobacco, and smokeless tobacco to anyone younger than age 18; the advertising restrictions were struck down by a federal district court, but the decision is under appeal by the government. The scope of the FDA's jurisdiction over tobacco, including regulation as a drug delivery device, remained unsettled as of the summer of 1997.

Health Resources and Services Administration (HRSA)
Founded: 1982. Headquarters: Rockville, MD. Purpose: To make essential primary care services accessible to the poor, uninsured, geographically isolated, and others who are severely underserved by the private health care system. It helps assist health providers meet the needs of the underserved by keeping pace with changes in health care, including managed care; provides primary care services to the working poor and uninsured through community and migrant health centers; and attends to the special health care needs of people with chronic health needs, minorities, and those living along the U.S. border with Mexico.

Holistic Dental Association (HAD)
Founded: 1980. Headquarters: Oklahoma City, OK. Purpose: To promote a holistic approach to better dental care for patients. To expand techniques, medications, and philosophies that pertain to extractions, anesthetics, fillings, crowns, and orthodontics. To encourage use of homeopathic medications, acupuncture, cranial osteopathy, nutritional techniques and physical therapy in addition to conventional treatments.

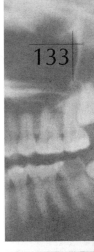

Indian Health Service (IHS)
Founded: 1955. Headquarters: Rockville, MD. Purpose: To raise the health status of American Indians and Alaskan Natives to the highest possible level. It facilitates and assists Indian tribes in coordinating health planning, in obtaining and using health resources available through federal, state, and local programs, and providing comprehensive health care services, including hospital and ambulatory medical care, preventive and rehabilitative services, and development of community sanitation facilities.

Institute of Medicine (IOM)
Founded: 1970. Headquarters: Washington, DC. Purpose: To serve as a component within the National Academy of Sciences to enlist distinguished members of the appropriate professions in the examination of policy matters pertaining to the health of the public. The IOM acts under both the academy's 1863 congressional charter responsibility to be an advisor to the federal government and its own initiative in identifying issues of medical care, research, and education. The IOM accomplishes its mission to advance scientific knowledge and health by providing objective, timely, and authoritative information to the government, the professions, and the public. Program operations in the IOM are Neuroscience and Behavioral Health; the Board on Children, Youth, and Families; Board on International Health; Food and Nutrition Board (FNB); Health Care Services; Health Promotion and Disease Prevention (includes AIDS Program); Health Sciences Policy; Medical Follow-up-Agency; National Cancer Policy Board (a joint board with the Commission Life Sciences); and Office of Health Policy Programs and Fellowships.

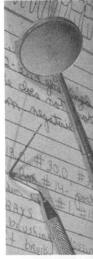

International Academy of Oral Medicine and Toxicology (IAOMT)
Founded: 1984. Headquarters: Orlando, FL. Purpose: To encourage, sponsor, and disseminate scientific research on the biocompatibility of materials used in dentistry; to offer educational programs; and to maintain speakers' bureau.

National Association of Dental Assistants (NADA)
Founded: 1974. Headquarters: Falls Church, VA. Purpose: To add to the professional stature of dental assistants through continuing education and to provide its members with benefits which are normally limited to specialized professional and fraternal groups. A job exchange service for dental assistants is also provided.

National Association of Dental Laboratories (NADL)
Founded: 1951. Headquarters: Alexandria, VA. Purpose: To provide management seminars and a basic laboratory technician's training program. Offers business and personal insurance programs, hazardous materials training program, an infectious disease prevention training program, business management and technical education programs. Serves commercial dental laboratories, industry manufacturers and suppliers, and schools of dental technology.

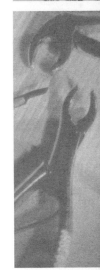

National Board for Certification in Dental Laboratories (CDL)
Founded: 1979. Headquarters: Alexandria, VA. Purpose: To provide certification and recognition of dental laboratories that demonstrate and document compliance with standards set by the industry. Serves certified dental laboratories, including commercial and private dental laboratories and dental or dental technology schools.

National Board for Certification in Dental Technology (NBC)
Founded: 1958. Headquarters: Alexandria, VA. Purpose: To establish standards and develop and conduct examinations; to certify dental technicians with formal education in dental technology and a minimum of three years' experience.

National Commission for Certifying Agencies (NCCA)
Founded: 1977. Headquarters: Washington, DC. Purpose: To help ensure the health, safety and welfare of the public through the accreditation of certification organizations that assess professional competence. NCCA is the accrediting body of the National Organization for Competency Assurance.

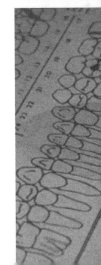

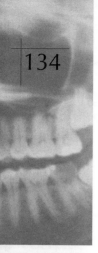
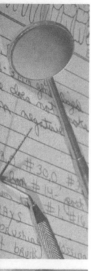
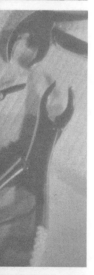
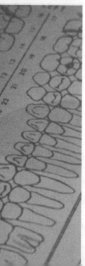

National Council in Measurement in Education (NCME)

Founded: About 1980. Headquarters: Washington, DC. Purpose: To advance the science of measurement in the field of education, to improve measurement instruments and procedures for their administration, scoring, interpretation and use, and to improve applications of measurement in assessment of individual and evaluations of educational programs.

National Dental Assistants Association (NDAA)

Founded: 1964. Headquarters: Washington, DC. Purpose: To encourage education and certification among dental assistants and to conduct clinics and workshops. It is an auxiliary of the National Dental Association.

National Dental Association (NDA)

Founded: 1913. Headquarters: Washington, DC. Purpose: To foster the provision of quality dental care to the unserved and underserved public and to promote knowledge of the art and science of dentistry; to foster the integration of minority dental health care providers in the profession; to promote dentistry as a viable career for minorities through scholarship and support programs; and to advocate the inclusion of dental care services in health care programs on local, state, and national levels.

National Institutes of Health (NIH)

Founded: 1887. Headquarters: Bethesda, MD. Purpose: To serve as the principal biomedical research agency of the federal government, with a mission to apply science in the pursuit of knowledge to improve human health conditions. NIH seeks to expand fundamental knowledge about the nature and behavior of living systems, to apply that knowledge to extend the health of human lives, and to reduce the burdens resulting from disease and disability. The NIH supports biomedical and behavioral research domestically and abroad, conducts research in its own laboratories and clinics, trains researchers, and promotes the acquisition and distribution of medical knowledge.

National Medical and Dental Association (NMDA)

Founded: 1910. Headquarters: Maspeth, NY. Purpose: To offer specialized education; to maintain a speakers' bureau and a hall of fame; and to provide a social organization for Polish-American professionals interested in preserving their heritage. Serves physicians, dentists, and lawyers of Polish extraction.

National Organization for Competency Assurance (NOCA)

Founded: 1977. Headquarters: Washington, DC. Purpose: To foster public awareness and acceptance of private-sector credentialing as an alternative to licensure and to promote nonlicensed but certified practitioners as a means to achieving high quality and cost containment. Serves nonprofit organizations conducting certification programs for occupations and professionals and for trade associations representing these professionals.

Occupational Safety and Health Administration (OSHA)

Founded: 1970. Headquarters: Washington, DC. Purpose: To develop and promulgate occupational safety and health standards; develop and issue regulations; conduct investigations and inspections to determine compliance; and to issue citations and propose penalties for noncompliance with safety and health standards. OSHA is charged with supporting the Occupational Safety and Health Act of 1970.

Organization for Safety and Asepsis Procedures (OSAP)

Founded: 1984. Headquarters: Annapolis, MD. Purpose: To promote infection control and related science-based health and safety policies and practices.

Union of American Physicians and Dentists (UAPD)

Founded: 1972. Headquarters: Oakland, CA. Purpose: To ensure reasonable compensation for physicians commensurate with their training, skill, and the responsibility they bear for their patients. Serves state federations made up of 10,000 physicians and dentists, self-employed or employed by hospitals, teaching institutions, counties, and municipalities.

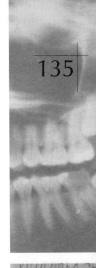

Administrative Secretary
Board of Dental Examiners of Alabama
5346 Stadium Trace Parkway, Ste. 112,
Hoover, AL 35224
Phone: 205/985-7267
Fax: 256/533-4690
www.dentalboard.org

Licensing Examiner
Alaska State Board of Dental Examiners
Division of Occupational Licensure
P.O. Box 110806
Juneau, AK 99811-0806
Phone: 907/465-2534
Fax: 907/465-2974
www.commerce.state.ak.us/occ

Executive Director
Arizona State Board of Dental Examiners
5060 N. 19th Ave. #406
Phoenix, AZ 85015
Phone: 602/242-1492
Fax: 602/242-1445
www.azdentalboard.org

Executive Director
Arkansas State Board of Dental Examiners
101 E. Capitol, Suite 111
Little Rock, AR 72201
Phone: 501/682-2085
Fax: 501/682-3543
www.asbde.org

Executive Officer
Dental Board of California
Committee on Dental Auxiliaries
1428 Howe Avenue, Suite 58
Sacramento, CA 95825
Phone: 916/263-2595
Fax: 916/263-2709
www.dbc.ca.gov or www.comda.ca.gov

Program Administrator
Colorado State Board of Dental Examiners
1560 Broadway, Suite 1310
Denver, CO 80202
Phone: 303/894-7758
Fax: 303/894-7764
www.dora.state.co.us/Dental

Health Program Supervisor
Connecticut State Dental Commission/
Dept. Of Public Health
410 Capitol Ave., MS #12 APP
P.O. Box 340308
Hartford, CT 06134
Phone: 860/509-8388
Fax: 860/509-8457
www.oralhealth.state.ct.us/index.html

Administrator
Delaware Department of Public Health/
Health Systems Management
417 Federal Street
Dover, DE 19901
Phone: 302/744-4700
Fax: 302/739-2711
www.state.de.us/research/profreg/dental.htm

Health License Specialist
Department of Health
DC Board of Dentistry
717 14th St. NW
Suite 600
Washington, DC 20005
Phone: 202/724-4900
Fax: 202/727-8471
www.dchealth.dc.gov

Executive Director
Florida Board of Dentistry
4052 Bald Cypress Way—Bin C08
Tallahassee, FL 32399
Phone: 850/245-4474
Fax: 850/921-5389
www.doh.state.fl.us/mqa

Executive Director
Georgia Board of Dentistry
237 Coliseum Drive
Macon, GA 31217
Phone: 478/207-1686
Fax: 478/207-1685
www.sos.state.ga.us/plb/dentistry/

Executive Officer
Hawaii State Board of Dental Examiners—
Dept. of Commerce and Consumer Affairs
P.O. Box 3469
Honolulu, HI 96801
Phone: 808/586-3000
Fax: 808/586-2874
www.hawaii.gov/dcca/pvl/areas_dentist.html

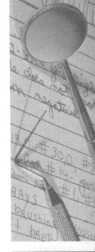

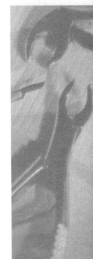

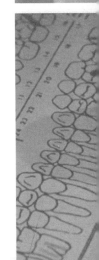

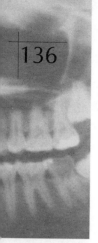

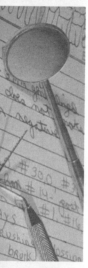

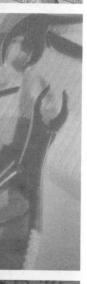

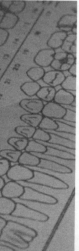

Administrator
Idaho State Board of Dentistry
708 1/2 W. Franklin Street
Boise, ID 83720-0021
Phone: 208/334-2369
Fax: 208/334-3247
www2.state.id.us/isbd

Administrator
**Illinois State Board of Dentistry—Dept.
of Professional Regulation & Education**
320 W. Washington, 3rd Floor
Springfield, IL 62786
Phone: 217/782-8566
Fax: 217/782-7645
www.dpr.state.il.us/WHO/dent.asp

Administrator
**Indiana State Dept. of Health/
Division of Medical Radiology Services**
2 Meridian Street, 5F
Indianapolis, IN 46204
Phone: 317/233-7565
Fax: 317/233-7154
www.in.gov/hpb/boards/isbd

Executive Director
Iowa Board of Dental Examiners
400 SW 8th St., Suite D
Des Moines, IA 50309-4687
Phone: 515/281-5157
Fax: 515/281-7969
www.state.ia.us/dentalboard/

Administrative Secretary
Kansas Dental Board
900 SW Jackson
Room 564-S
Topeka, KS 66612
Phone: 785/296-6400
Fax: 785/296-3116
www.accesskansas.org/kdb

Executive Director
Kentucky Board of Dentistry
10101 Linn Station Rd. #540
Louisville, KY 40223
Phone: 502/423-0573
Fax: 502/423-1239
http://dentistry.ky.gov

Executive Director
Louisiana State Board of Dentistry
365 Canal Street, Suite 2680
New Orleans, LA 70130
Phone: 504/568-8574
Fax: 504/568-8598
www.lsbd.org

Executive Secretary
Maine Board of Dental Examiners
Two Bangor Street
Augusta, ME 04333-0143
Phone: 207/287-3333
Fax: 207/287-8140
www.mainedental.org

Adminstrator
**Maryland State Board of Dental
Examiners**
The Benjamin Rush Bldg.
Spring Grove Hospital Center
Wade Avenue
Baltimore, MD 21228
Phone: 410/402-8500
Fax: 410/402-8505
www.dhmh.state.md.us/dental

Executive Director
Massachusets Board of Dentistry
239 Causeway Street, Suite 500
Boston, MA 02114
Phone: 617/727-0084
Fax: 617/727-2197
www.state.ma.us/reg/boards/dn

Licensing Manager
Michigan Board of Dentistry
P.O. Box 30670
Lansing, MI 48909-8170
Phone: 517/335-1752
Fax: 517/373-2179
www.michigan.gov/healthlicense

Executive Director
Minnesota Board of Dentistry
2829 University Ave., SE
Suite 450
Minneapolis, MN 55414-3246
Phone: 612/617-2250
Fax: 612/617-2260
www.dentalboard.state.mn.us

Executive Director
**Mississippi State Board of Dental
Examiners**
600 East Amite Street, Suite 100
Jackson, MS 39201-2801
Phone: 601/944-9622
Fax: 601/944-9624
www.msbde.state.ms.us

Executive Director
Missouri Dental Board
3605 Missouri Blvd.
P.O. Box 1367
Jefferson City, MO 65102-1367
Phone: 573/751-0040
Fax: 573-751-8216
http://pr.mo.gov/dental.asp

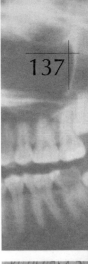

Administrator
Montana Board of Dentistry
301 S. Park, 4th Fl
Helena, MT 59620-0513
Phone: 406/841-2390
Fax: 406/841-2305
www.discoveringmontana.com/dli/den

Credentialing Coordinator
Nebraska Board of Dentistry
Credentialing Division
P.O. Box 94986
Lincoln, NE 68509-4986
Phone: 402/471-2118
Fax: 402/471-3577
www.hhs.state.ne.us/crl/medical/dent/
dentist/dentist.html

Executive Director
Nevada Board of Dental Examiners
2295 Renaissance Drive, Suite B
Las Vegas, NV 89119
Phone: 702/486-7044/800-DDS-EXAM
Fax: 702/486-7046
www.nvdentalboard.org/index.html

Executive Secretary
New Hampshire Board of Dental
Examiners
2 Industrial Park Drive
Concord, NH 03301-8520
Phone: 603/271-4561
Fax: 603/271-6702
www.state.nh.us/dental

Executive Director
New Jersey State Board of Dentistry
124 Halsey Street, 6th Floor
6th Floor
P.O. Box 45005
Newark, NJ 07101
Phone: 973/504-6405
Fax: 973/273-8075
www.state.nj.us/lps/ca/
medical.htm#den3

Administrator
New Mexico Board of
Dental Health Care
P.O.Box 25101
Santa Fe, NM 87504-5101
Phone: 505/476-4680
Fax: 505/476-4545
www.rld.state.nm.us/b&c/dental/
index.htm

Executive Secretary
New York State Board for Dentistry
89 Washington Avenue
2nd Floor West Wing
Albany, NY 12234
Phone: 518/474-3817 x270
Fax: 518/473-6995
www.op.nysed.gov/dent.htm

Licensing Coordinator
North Carolina State Board of Dental
Examiners
15100 Westin Parkway
Suite 101
Cary, NC 27513-2129
Phone: 919/678-8223
Fax: 919/678-8472
www.ncdentalboard.org

Executive Director
North Dakota Board of Dentistry
P.O. Box 7246
Bismarck, ND 58507-7246
Phone: 701/258-8600
Fax: 701/224-9824
www.nddentalboard.org

Executive Director
Ohio State Dental Board
77 S. High Street
18th Floor
Columbus, OH 43215-6135
Phone: 614/466-2580
Fax: 614/752-8995
www.state.oh.us/den

Executive Director
Oklahoma Board of Dentistry
201 NE 38th Terrace
Suite 2
Oklahoma City, OK 73105
Phone: 405/524-9037
Fax: 405/524-2223
www.dentist.state.ok.us/

Executive Director
Oregon Board of Dentistry
1600 SW 4th Ave.
Suite 770
Portland, OR 97201
Phone: 503/229-5520
Fax: 503/229-6606
www.oregondentistry.org

Board Administrator
Pennsylvania State Board of Dentistry
P.O. Box 2649
Harrisburg, PA 17105
Phone: 717/783-7162
Fax: 717/782-7769
www.dos.state.pa.us/dent

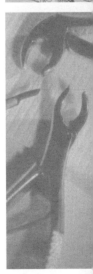

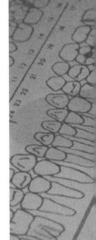

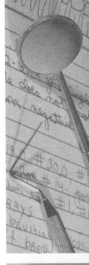

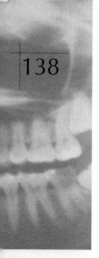

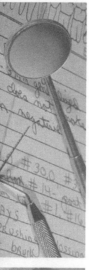

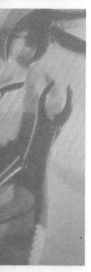

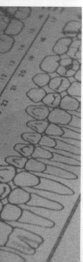

Director, Examining Boards
Puerto Rico Board of Dental Examiners
Department of Health
Call Box 10200
San Juan, PR 00908
Phone: 787/725-8161
Fax: 809-7257903

Administrator
Rhode Island State Board of Examiners in
Dentistry
3 Capitol Hill, Room 104
Providence, RI 02908-5097
Phone: 401/222-1392
Fax: 401/222-1272
www.health.state.ri.us/hsr/professions/
dental.htm

Executive Director
South Carolina State Board of Dentistry
P.O. Box 11329
Columbia, SC 29211-1329
Phone: 803/896-4599
Fax: 803/896-4596
www.llr.state.sc.us/pol/dentistry/
default.htm

Executive Secretary
South Dakota State Board of Dentistry
P.O. Box 1037
106 W. Capitol
Pierre, SD 57501-1037
Phone: 605/224-1282
Fax: 605/224-7426
www.state.sd.us/doh/dentistry

Administrator
Tennessee Board of Dentistry
1st Floor, Cordell Hull Bldg.
425 5th Avenue, North
Nashville, TN 37247-1010
Phone: 800/778-4123 ext. 24721
Fax: 615/532-5369
www2.state.tn.us/health/Boards/Dentistry/

Executive Director
Texas State Board of Dental Examiners
333 Guadalupe Street, Twr. 3,
Suite 800
Austin, TX 78701
Phone: 512/463-6400
Fax: 512/463-7452
www.tsbde.state.tx.us

Bureau Manager
Utah Dentists and Dental Hygienists
Licensing Board
P.O. Box 146741
Salt Lake City, UT 84114-6741
Phone: 801/530-6740
Fax: 801/530-6511
www.dopl.utah.gov/licensing/dental.html

Staff Assistant/Executive Secretary
Vermont State Board of Dental
Examiners–Secretary of State's Office
26 Terrance Street, Drawer 09
Montpelier, VT 05609-1106
Phone: 802/828-2390
Fax: 802/828-2465
www.vtprofessionals.org/opr1/dentists/

Executive Director
Virginia Board of Dentistry
6603 W. Broad St. 5th Floor
Richmond, VA 23230-1712
Phone: 804/662-9906
Fax: 804/662-7246
www.dhp.virginia.gov/dentistry/
default.htm

Executive Assistant
Virgin Islands Board of Dental
Examiners–Department of Health
48 Sugar Estate
St. Thomas, USVI 00802
Phone: 340/774-0117
Fax: 340/777-4001

Executive Director
Washington State Dental Health Care
Quality Assurance Commission
310 Isreal Road SE
P.O. Box 47860
Olympia, WA 98504-7867
Phone: 360/236-4700
Fax: 360/753-0675
www.doh.wa.gov/A-Z.htm

Administrator
West Virginia Board of Dental Examiners
207 Heber Street
Beckley, WV 25801
Phone: 877/914-8266
Fax: 304/253-9454
www.wvdentalboard.org

Administrator
Wisconsin Dentistry Examining Board
P.O. Box 8935
1400 E. Washington Ave.
Madison , WI 53708-8935
Phone: 608/266-2811
Fax: 608/267-0644
http://drl.wi.gov/boards/den/index.htm

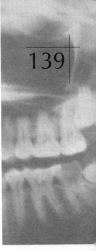

Board Administrator
Wyoming Board of Dental Examiners
2020 Carey Ave.
Suite 201
Cheyenne, WY 82002
Phone: 307/777-6529
Fax: 307/777-3508
http://plboards.state.wy.us/dental/
index.asp

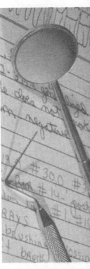

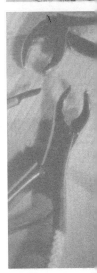

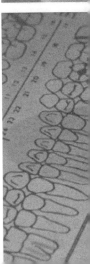

NOTES